Esophageal Cancer

Guest Editor

GUY D. ESLICK, PhD, MMedSc
(Clin Epi), MMedStat

GASTROENTEROLOGY
CLINICS OF NORTH AMERICA

www.gastro.theclinics.com

March 2009 • Volume 38 • Number 1

SAUNDERS an imprint of ELSEVIER, Inc.

W.B. SAUNDERS COMPANY

A Division of Elsevier Inc.

Elsevier Inc. • 1600 John F. Kennedy Blvd., Suite 1800 • Philadelphia, Pennsylvania 19103-2899

http://www.theclinics.com

GASTROENTEROLOGY CLINICS OF NORTH AMERICA Volume 38, Number 1
March 2009 ISSN 0889-8553, ISBN-13: 978-1-4377-0477-8, ISBN-10: 1-4377-0477-8

Editor: Kerry Holland

Gastroenterology Clinics of North America (ISSN 0889-8553) is published quarterly by Elsevier Inc., 360 Park Avenue South, New York, NY 10010-1710. Months of issue are March, June, September, and December. Business and Editorial Offices: 1600 John F. Kennedy Blvd., Suite 1800, Philadelphia, PA 19103-2899. Customer Service Office: 6277 Sea Harbor Drive, Orlando, FL 32887-4800. Periodicals postage paid at New York, NY and additional mailing offices. Subscription prices are $256.00 per year (US individuals), $131.00 per year (US students), $385.00 per year (US institutions), $282.00 per year (Canadian individuals), $469.00 per year (Canadian institutions), $355.00 per year (international individuals), $181.00 per year (international students), and $469.00 per year (international institutions). Foreign air speed delivery is included in all *Clinics* subscription prices. All prices are subject to change without notice. **POSTMASTER:** Send address changes to *Gastroenterology Clinics of North America*, Elsevier Periodicals Customer Service 11830 Westline Industrial Drive, St. Louis, MO 63146. **Customer Service: 1-800-654-2452 (US). From outside the United States, call 1-314-453-7041. Fax: 1-314-453-5170. E-mail: journalscustomerservice-usa@elsevier.com (for print support) or journalsonline support-usa@elsevier.com (for online support).**

Reprints. For copies of 100 or more, of articles in this publication, please contact the Commercial Reprints Department, Elsevier Inc., 360 Part Avenue South, New York, New York 10010-1710. Tel. (212) 633-3813, Fax: (212) 462-1935, e-mail: reprints@elsevier.com.

Gastroenterology Clinics of North America is also published in Italian by Il Pensiero Scientifico Editore, Rome, Italy; and in Portuguese by Interlivros Edicoes Ltda., Rua Commandante Coelho 1085, 21250 Cordovil, Rio de Janeiro, Brazil.

Gastroenterology Clinics of North America is covered in *MEDLINE/PubMed (Index Medicus), Excerpta Medica, Current Contents/Clinical Medicine, Science Citation Index, ISI/BIOMED,* and *BIOSIS*.

Printed and bound by CPI Group (UK) Ltd, Croydon, CR0 4YY

Transferred to Digital Print 2011

Contributors

GUEST EDITOR

GUY D. ESLICK, PhD, MMedSc (Clin Epi), MMedStat
Honorary Associate, Department of Public Health, School of Public Health, The University of Sydney, Sydney, New South Wales, Australia; Research Fellow, Harvard School of Public Health, Department of Epidemiology, Boston, Massachusetts

AUTHORS

CHRISTIAN C. ABNET, PhD, MPH
Division of Cancer Epidemiology and Genetics, National Cancer Institute Bethesda, Maryland

JAFFER A. AJANI, MD
Professor of Medicine, Department of GI Medical Oncology, The University of Texas M.D. Anderson Cancer Center, Houston, Texas

ALAN BRIJBASSIE, MD
Internal Medicine Resident, Carilion Clinic, Roanoke, Virgina

STEPHEN D. CASSIVI, MD, MSc
Associate Professor of Surgery, Department of Surgery, Division of General Thoracic Surgery, Mayo Clinic, Rochester, Minnesota

WINSON Y. CHEUNG, MD
Medical Oncology and Hematology, Department of Medicine, Princess Margaret Hospital/Ontario Cancer Institute, University of Toronto, Toronto, Ontario, Canada; Department of Epidemiology, Harvard School of Public Health, Boston, Massachusetts

WONG-HO CHOW, PhD
Division of Cancer Epidemiology and Genetics, National Cancer Institute, Bethesda, Maryland

SANFORD M. DAWSEY, MD
Division of Cancer Epidemiology and Genetics, National Cancer Institute, Bethesda, Maryland

GUY D. ESLICK, PhD, MMedSc (Clin Epi), MMedStat
Honorary Associate, Department of Public Health, School of Public Health, The University of Sydney, Sydney, Australia; Research Fellow, Program in Molecular and Genetic Epidemiology, Harvard School of Public Health, Boston, Massachusetts

DAVID H. ILSON, MD, PhD
Gastrointestinal Oncology Service, Department of Medicine, Memorial Sloan-Kettering Cancer Center, New York, New York

FARIN KAMANGAR, MD, PhD
Division of Cancer Epidemiology and Genetics, National Cancer Institute, Bethesda, Maryland

GEOFFREY Y. KU, MD
Ludwig Center for Cancer Immunotherapy, Memorial Sloan-Kettering Cancer Center, New York, New York

GEOFFREY LIU, MD, MSc
Medical Oncology and Hematology, Department of Medicine; and Applied Molecular Oncology, Medical Biophysics, Princess Margaret Hospital/Ontario Cancer Institute, University of Toronto, Toronto, Ontario, Canada; Departments of Environmental and Occupational Medicine and Epidemiology, Harvard School of Public Health, Boston, Massachusetts

VAL J. LOWE, MD
Professor of Radiology, Director of PET/CT Imaging, Department of Radiology, Division of Nuclear Medicine, Mayo Clinic, Rochester, Minnesota

ELIZABETH A. MONTGOMERY, MD
Professor, Department of Pathology, The Johns Hopkins Medical Institutions, Baltimore, Maryland

YVONNE ROMERO, MD
Associate Professor of Medicine, Division of Gastroenterology and Hepatology; Department of Otolaryngology, Mayo Clinic, Rochester, Minnesota

JENNIFER R. SCUDIERE, MD
Faculty Assistant, Department of Pathology, The Johns Hopkins Medical Institutions, Baltimore, Maryland

VANESSA M. SHAMI, MD
Director of Endoscopic Ultrasonography, and Assistant Professor, Department of Medicine, Division of Gastroenterology, University of Virginia Digestive Health Center of Excellence, Charlottesville, Virginia

SANDRA TOMASZEK, MD
Research Fellow, Division of General Thoracic Surgery, Mayo Clinic, Rochester, Minnesota

YUTAKA TOMIZAWA, MD
Barrett's Esophagus Unit, Division of Gastroenterology and Hepatology, Mayo Clinic, Rochester, Minnesota

KENNETH K. WANG, MD
Professor of Medicine, Director, Barrett's Esophagus Unit, Division of Gastroenterology and Hepatology, Mayo Clinic; Barrett's Esophagus Unit, Alfred Main, Gastroenterology Diagnostic Unit, St. Mary's Hospital, Rochester, Minnesota

TAIXIANG WU, MD
Professor, Chinese Clinical Trial Registry, Chinese Cochrane Centre, Chinese EBM Centre, INCLEN Local Training Center in West China Hospital, Sichuan University, Chengdu, China

XUNZHE YANG, MSc
Chinese Cochrane Centre, Chinese EBM Centre, West China Hospital, Sichuan
University, Chengdu, China

HARRY H. YOON, MD, MHS
Assistant Professor, Division of Medical Oncology, Mayo Clinic, Rochester, Minnesota

XIAOXI ZENG, MSc
Chinese Cochrane Centre, Chinese EBM Centre, West China Hospital, Sichuan
University, Chengdu, China

Contents

The history of esophageal cancer dates back to ancient Egyptian times, circa 3000 BC. Since then, the progress in the diagnosis and treatment of esophageal cancer has been steady. Over the last few centuries there have been advancements in the visualization and removal of these lesions, but with no real overall impact on survival rates. The twenty-first century is the time to make major progress in not only improving survival rates, but also in diagnosing esophageal cancer in the very early stages.

The epidemiology of esophageal cancer has radically changed in the last fifty-years in the Western world. Changes in the predominant type of squamous cell carcinoma to adenocarcinoma, disparities between different ethnicities, and the exponential increase in incidence rates of adenocarcinoma have established esophageal cancer as a major public health problem requiring urgent attention.

This article reviews the environmental risk factors and predisposing conditions for the two main histologic types of esophageal cancer. Tobacco smoking, excessive alcohol consumption, drinking maté, low intake of fresh fruits and vegetables, achalasia, and low socioeconomic status increase the risk of esophageal squamous cell carcinoma. Results of investigations on other potential risk factors, including opium consumption, intake of hot drinks, eating pickled vegetables, poor oral health, and exposure to human papillomavirus, polycyclic aromatic hydrocarbons, *N*-nitroso compounds, acetaldehyde, and fumonisins are discussed. Gastroesophageal reflux, obesity, tobacco smoking, hiatal hernia, achalasia, and, probably, absence of H pylori in the stomach increase the risk of esophageal adenocarcinoma. Results of studies investigating other factors are also discussed.

The incidence of esophageal cancer, especially esophageal adenocarcinoma, is increasing and its high mortality rate is a notable fact. Improving survival rates of this disease depend on earlier detection through screening and surveillance; however, standard diagnostic modalities, such as endoscopy with biopsy, have several limitations as screening tools, including low negative predictive value and relatively high cost. Recently developed biomarkers such as FISH and improved imaging techniques, may help overcome current problems and provide improved screening and surveillance for esophageal cancer.

Investigations into inherited genetic variations in the DNA code (known as polymorphisms) in the field of oncology have provided preliminary support for an association with cancer risks and outcomes. Early studies have highlighted several genes with this potential predictive and prognostic power. However, these studies have had methodological limitations and have produced inconsistent results, making impractical as yet the routine evaluation of such genetic polymorphisms in general clinical practice. Continued research in this area is essential if we are to be able to soon use genetic polymorphisms to better select patients for targeted anticancer interventions. This review discusses the role of genetic polymorphisms and their association with esophageal cancer risk and prognosis. The article also highlights future directions in this new, emerging field of molecular epidemiology.

Esophageal malignancy is a major source of morbidity and mortality, despite the recently increased attention to screening and early detection. Prognosis for esophageal cancer remains grim, with advanced tumor stage and lymph node metastases conferring even graver outcomes. Several studies have demonstrated that the addition of preoperative neoadjuvant chemoradiotherapy may improve survival in patients with locally advanced tumor (T3) disease or local lymph node metastases. It is here that endoscopic ultrasonography finds its niche in the precise staging of these tumors and the subsequent use of stage-dependent treatment protocols.

THE CLINICS ARE NOW AVAILABLE ONLINE!

Access your subscription at:
www.theclinics.com

Preface

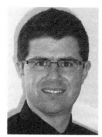

Guy D. Eslick, PhD, MMedSc (Clin Epi), MMedStat
Guest Editor

It is with tremendous optimism that I welcome you to this issue of *Gastroenterology Clinics of North America*, which is devoted to esophageal cancer. Esophageal cancer is on the rise in terms of incidence in the Western world, and survival rates have not improved much in the last 30 years. This lack of progress in survival rates is mainly because, unfortunately, most individuals only develop symptoms after the cancer has already metastasized to other organs, by which time a cure is usually out of the question. Esophageal cancer is a devastating disease. As Lyman A. Brewer IIII said, "No patients with malignancy are more miserable than those suffering unrelieved malignant obstruction of the esophagus, because they ultimately die of slow starvation" (*Am J Surg* 1980:139:730–43). Esophageal cancer is a major public health problem, and the time has come for funding bodies (in particular, cancer organizations) to take greater notice and dedicate increased funding to all aspects of esophageal cancer research.

The topics selected for this issue of *Gastroenterology Clinics of North America* have been chosen for two reasons. The first is to fill gaps in knowledge. Thus, new information is presented on cutting-edge topics, such as genetic polymorphisms, and on topics unfamiliar to many in the field, such as the use of Chinese herbal medicines. The second reason is to provide the latest information on advances in such areas as clinical pathology, epidemiology, positron emission tomography, ultrasonography, and environmental causes of esophageal cancer. It has been a true pleasure reading and editing this outstanding collection of articles written by leading authorities in the field.

As I was preparing for this issue, I found some interesting trivia about people who had developed esophageal cancer. Two actors had made comments about what they "jokingly" thought might have been the cause of their esophageal cancer. The first was Humphrey Bogart (1899–1957), who was diagnosed with esophageal cancer in 1956. He was a heavy drinker and cigarette smoker. He had surgery that involved an esophagectomy, removal of two lymph nodes, and a rib, and he also had a course of postsurgical chemotherapy. He had radiation therapy due to recurrence of the cancer 6 months after surgery. He died at home after falling into a coma. His last words were: "I never should have switched from scotch to martinis." The second was Jack

doi:10.1016/j.gtc.2009.01.013
0889-8553/09/$ – see front matter © 2009 Elsevier Inc. All rights reserved.

gastro.theclinics.com

Soo (1917–1979), a Japanese-American actor who was cast in the 1970s television comedy *Barney Miller* as the laid-back, but very wry, Detective Nick Yemana, who was also responsible for making the awful coffee that everyone in the office had the misfortune to drink every day. Just before he was taken into the operating room before his death, his last words to his *Barney Miller* co-star Hal Linden were: "It must have been the coffee." Some other well-known people who had esophageal cancer include Japanese children's author Kenjiro Haitani (1934–2006); University of Miami basketball legend Dick Hickox (1938–2006); actor Makoto "Mako" Iwamatsu (1933–2006); Jaap Penraat (1918–2006), who helped 406 Jews escape the Holocaust; Texas Governor Ann Richards (1933–2006); and Larry Stewart (1948–2007), who anonymously gave away $100 bills to the needy each December as "Secret Santa."

I would like to thank the senior editor of *Gastroenterology Clinics of North America*, Kerry Holland, for her valuable advice, patience, and assistance in putting this issue into publication. I would also like to give special thanks to my wife, Enid, and our daughter, Marielle, for their love and support.

One of the main reasons for developing this issue on esophageal cancer was not only to update and educate, but more so to invigorate, not just those clinicians and researchers currently treating esophageal cancer patients or conducting medical research on esophageal cancer, but also those young investigators who want to make a difference in the lives of those with cancer. I strongly encourage you to come forward and join the battle against this devastating yet interesting disease.

Guy D. Eslick, PhD, MMedSc (Clin Epi), MMedStat
School of Public Health
The University of Sydney
Sydney, New South Wales
Australia

Harvard School of Public Health
Department of Epidemiology
677 Huntington Avenue
Building II, 2nd Floor, Room 209
Boston, MA 02115, USA

E-mail address:
geslick@hsph.harvard.edu

Dedication

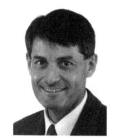

Philip G. McManis, MD

I would like to dedicate this issue of the *Gastroenterology Clinics of North America* to a colleague, Associate Professor Philip G. McManis, MD, who died peacefully of esophageal cancer on September 17 in 2004 at age 51 years (*Neurology* 2005;64:598–599). Philip possessed great charm, a fierce determination, an acute intelligence, and a fine sense of humor. He was widely loved and respected. He was a wonderful husband and father. He was a supreme physician. Many thousands of friends and patients are in his debt.

Philip had no risk factors for the development of esophageal cancer and had no gastrointestinal symptoms until 3 months before diagnosis. In an e-mail to a colleague, he said, "I noticed that bread would stick at the lower end of the esophagus, but thought little of that. About a month ago, it started getting worse and I began having to eat slowly to avoid painful esophageal spasms, so I thought I should get it checked out. Ten days ago, I had a gastroscopy, which showed a fungating lesion at the cardioesophageal junction, and a biopsy showed adenocarcinoma, moderately well differentiated. There was no other abnormality and no signs of Barrett's esophagus."

In a recent e-mail from Philip's wife Tamera, she poignantly describes Philip and his experience with esophageal cancer.

"Philip was truly amazing during his illness. I remember Philip consistently endeavored to make it easier for others, particularly his treating physicians, when they had to give him bad news (he was always several steps ahead of them)—he seemed literally to feel worse for them than he did about his condition and what he was ultimately facing. I remember toward the end, about 3 months before Philip died and he had had his dose of taxatere—by this stage the cancer had ravaged his body and the effects of the taxatere were equally less forgiving—he had a scan of his liver and although he hadn't seen the results, he pretty much knew his liver was riddled with metastases, and he knew if he were lucky, he may have a couple of months, but in true character, it was never really about him, it was about all those who he cared about: his patients, his colleagues, and his friends and family. He endured much pain throughout the 18-month illness—mainly because he didn't want medications to interfere with his capacity to continue to treat his patients, which of course he did up to a week before

Gastroenterol Clin N Am 38 (2009) xv–xvi
doi:10.1016/j.gtc.2009.01.002

he died. Philip pretty much slept sitting up because it was too painful to lie down. His stamina was staggering. He somehow managed to tote his portable EMG [electromyogram] machine around until the end; I distinctly remember the moment he set it down for the last time.

On a personal note, I don't know if the pain of losing Philip will ever disappear, but I know it will lessen with time. His love will be in my memories and they will grow richer and even more pleasant with time. I feel great comfort, too, knowing that Philip will be in the faces, character, and souls of our children who are a wonderful expression of the special union and bond that we had in this lifetime. What I have learned from this experience is that like Philip, we have to live each moment of each day to the maximum and try as best we can to express our love through caring. If we are able to do this, I think life's trip will be worth it. I think it is fitting that in Philip's death, he reminds us of what we need to do to make our lives worth living. That will be my tribute to Philip. If I had to summarize how we as a family approached Philip's illness and death, it would be simply that Philip helped us to go on living and we helped him to die, with dignity, with acceptance, and most of all with love."

Guy D. Eslick, PhD

Esophageal Cancer: A Historical Perspective

Guy D. Eslick, PhD, MMedSc (Clin Epi), MMedStat[a,b,*]

KEYWORDS

- Esophageal cancer • Adenocarcinoma • History
- Progress • Historical

In the history of esophageal cancer, the majority of initial discoveries were made in the nineteenth and twentieth centuries. However, the earliest mention of esophageal cancer appears to have come from Egypt around 3000 BC, and there were further reports from China around 2000 years ago. Then, between the sixteenth and nineteenth centuries, there were advancements in the visualization and removal of these lesions. In the twentieth century these techniques were improved upon, but with no real increase in survival rates. Currently, the technological instruments and treatment options available are amazing when compared with even 50 years ago, but the majority of cases are still diagnosed at late stage and there has been no substantial overall improvement in outcomes from this insidious disease. The literature is scattered and can be extremely difficult to locate; as such, this article focuses on a few key historical moments associated with esophageal cancer diagnosis and treatment. **Box 1** shows a historical timeline of esophageal cancer.

ANCIENT TIMES
Egypt

One of the first human written descriptions of disease states including the anatomy, physiology, pathology, and clinical observation was discovered in 1862 by American egyptologist Edwin Smith and is known as the "Smith Surgical Papyrus" (**Fig. 1**), which was dated to have been transcribed between 3000 and 2500 BC (see **Box 1**).[1] Although there is no specific mention of esophageal cancer in the papyrus, it is worth mentioning case 28 of the 48 cases recorded for historic interest, titled "A Gaping Wound of the Throat Penetrating the Gullet." The translation of the material, including headings used, is shown below:[2]

Guy D. Eslick is supported by The International Union Against Cancer and the American Cancer Society, with an International Fellowship for Beginning Investigators.

[a] School of Public Health, The University of Sydney, Sydney, New South Wales, Australia
[b] Program in Molecular and Genetic Epidemiology, Harvard School of Public Health, 677 Huntington Avenue, Building II, 2nd Floor, Room 209, Boston, MA 02115, USA
* Molecular and Genetic Epidemiology, Harvard School of Public Health, 677 Huntington Avenue, Building II, 2nd Floor, Room 209, Boston, MA 02115, USA.
E-mail address: geslick@hsph.harvard.edu

Gastroenterol Clin N Am 38 (2009) 1–15
doi:10.1016/j.gtc.2009.01.003
0889-8553/09/$ – see front matter. Crown Copyright © 2009 Published by Elsevier Inc. All rights reserved.

Box 1
Historical timeline of esophageal cancer

3000–2500 BC: "Smith Surgical Papyrus" describes repair of the "gullet" after perforation; however, no mention of cancer.

950 BC: The Greek terms for "esophagus" and "stomach" appear in Homeric literature.

AD 0–1: The Chinese describe "swallowing syndromes" caused by cancer.

131–200: Galen describes fleshy growths causing obstruction of the gullet.

11th Century: Avicenna discusses the causes of dysphagia, including tumor involvement.

1363: Chauliac describes foreign bodies in the esophagus.

1543: Vesalius describes the anatomy of the esophagus.

16th Century: J. Fernel writes of scirrhus and other tumors blocking the esophageal tube and causing difficulty in swallowing.

1592: Fabricius Aquapendente employs wax tampers to remove foreign bodies from the esophagus.

1674: T. Willis uses whale bone to dilate the esophagus.

1724: Boerhaave reports a case of spontaneous rupture of the esophagus.

1764: Ludlow describes a pharyngesophageal diverticulum.

1806: Bozzini develops an early endoscope using a mirror and reflected light from a candle in an attempt to see the upper esophagus.

1809: Pinel recommends the use of esophageal tubes to feed the insane.

1821: Purton describes a case of esophageal achalasia.

1822: Magendie notes that food is held up at the lower end of the esophagus, suggesting the presence of a sphincter.

1843: Switzer invents the esophageal dilators.

1844: The first recorded operation of esophagotomy for the relief of esophageal stricture by John Watson an American surgeon.

1857: Albrecht Theodor Von Middeldorpf, a Breslau surgeon, performs the first operation on a tumor of the esophagus.

1868: Kussmaul is the first to pass a lighted tube through the entire esophagus into the stomach.

1871: Billroth successfully resects and reanastomoses the cervical esophagus in dogs.

1872: First excision of the esophagus in man, performed by Christian Albert Theodor Billroth, an Austrian surgeon.

1877: Czerny is the first to successfully resect the cervical esophagus for carcinoma in human beings.

1881: Mikulicz studies the physiology of the esophagus.

1883: Esophageal motility in human beings is determined by H. Kronecker and S. Meltzer with pressure measurements of inserted balloons.

1886: J. Mikulicz treats esophageal carcinoma by resetion and plastic reconstruction.

1898: Rehn attempts resections of an esophageal carcinoma via right posterior mediastinotomy in two patients, unsuccessfully.

1901: Dobromysslow successfully performs the first intrathoracic resection and reanastomosis of the esophagus in dogs.

1905: Beck describes formations of a gastric tube from the greater curvature of the stomach, based on the gastroepiploic artery.

1907: Wendell describes transpleural resection of an esophageal carcinoma of the lower esophagus with lateral esophagogastrostomy in a lumen (patient dies the following day).

1908: Volecker successfully resects a carcinoma of the gastroesophageal junction with primary esophagogastrostomy via laparotomy.

1913: Zaaijer successfully resects a carcinoma of the cardia via an abdominothoracic approach.

1913: Torek, using a transthoracic approach, is the first to successfully resect an esophageal carcinoma.

1933: Oshawa resects the thoracic esophagus for carcinoma with immediate esophagogastrostomy (8 of 18 patients survive).

1938: Adams is the first surgeon in the United States to perform transthoracic esophageal resection with immediate esophagogastrostomy.

1946: Ivor Lewis introduces esophagectomy and esophagogastrostomy through a right thoractomy.

1947: Sweet completes 212 resections for esophageal carcinoma (17% operative mortality and 8% 5-year survival).

1950: N.R. Barrett reviews what is now called Barrett's esophagus, previously reported by W. Tileston (1906), A. Lyall (1937), and P.R. Allison (1943). The complication of adenocarcinoma is noted by B.C. Morson and J.R. Belcher (1952).

1954: C.A. Clarke and R.B. McConnell connect the occurrence of tylosis and carcinoma of the esophagus.

1954: L.R. Celestin develops an esophageal tube widely used for the relief of malignant dysphagia.

1963: Logan describes 853 resections for esophageal carcinoma (29% operative mortality).

1970: C.F. Pope determines the histologic changes of reflux esophagitis obtained on endoscopy.

1971: A. Vanderwonden document the dysplastic transformation of Barrett's esophagus.

1978: Orringer and Sloan revive the technique of Gray Turner's "esophagectomy without thoracotomy."

1982: D. Fleischer employs endoscopic laser therapy to palliate cases of esophageal carcinoma.

1984: Leichman and colleagues at Wayne State University combine 3,000 cGy with two cycles of 5-FU and cisplatin preoperatively in 21 patients with squamous cell carcinoma of the esophagus (37% pathologic complete response; operative mortality 27%).

1997: Multiple phase III randomized trials fail to show significant survival benefit for neoadjuvant multimodality therapy.

21st Century: New endoscopy techniques, new types of chemotherapy, advances in radiological instruments and improvements in surveillance.

Adapted from Lee RB, Miller JI. Esophagectomy for cancer. Surg Clin North Am 1997;77:1171, with permission.

Examination
If thou examinest a man having a gaping wound in his piercing through to his gullet; if he drinks water he chokes (and) it come out of the mouth of his wound; it is greatly inflamed, so that he develops fever from it; thou shouldst draw together that wound with stitching.

Diagnosis
Thou shouldst say concerning him: "One having a wound in his throat, piercing through to his gullet. An ailment with which I will contend."

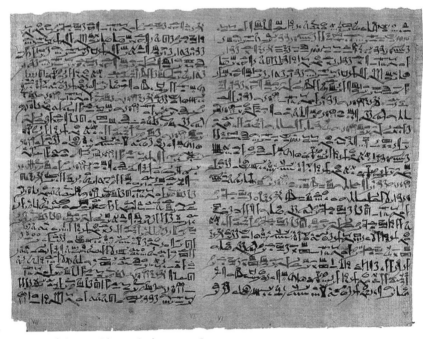

Fig. 1. Part of the "Smith surgical papyrus."

First treatment
Thou shouldst bind it with fresh meat the first day. Thou shouldst treat it afterwards with grease, honey, (and) lint every day, until he recovers.

Second examination
If, however, thou findst him continuing to have fever from that wound.

Second treatment
Thou shouldst apply dry lint in the mouth of his wound, (and) moor (him) at his mooring stakes until he recovers.

Roman Empire

Galen (**Fig. 2**), a famous Roman physician and philosopher who lived around AD 125–200, was purportedly the most accomplished medical researcher of the Roman period. His published work on the causes of symptoms mentions the possibility of a fleshy growth partially or entirely obstructing the passage of food down the gullet.

Persian Empire

Avicenna (AD 980–1037), who is regarded as the father of early modern medicine, also wrote about esophageal cancer (**Fig. 3**). In one of his published works, titled *The Canon of Medicine* published in 1025, he suggested that dysphagia was the most important symptom of tumors (apostema) of the esophagus.

China

The earliest reports of esophageal cancer in China appeared over 2000 years ago and were referred to as "Ye Ge," which means dysphagia and belching.[3] Reports of the

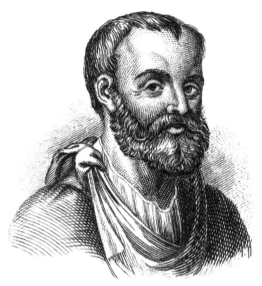

Fig. 2. Galen, the physician of the Roman Empire.

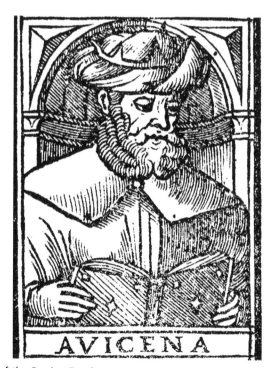

Fig. 3. Avicenna, of the Persian Empire.

disease have been recorded in traditional Chinese medical texts, with some of the authors suggesting that these particular cancers were a result of "heavy indulgence of heated liquors."[3] Moreover, others stated that esophageal cancer was more commonly seen in the elderly and rarely occurred in young people. In Henan Province, historical records report "dysphagia syndromes" among the inhabitants approximately 2000 years ago. In addition, in Linxian there had been a condition called "ge shi bing" (hard-of-swallowing disease), which has been present for several generations. Esophageal cancer was so feared in ancient times in this region that a temple was erected and it was known as the "Houwang Miao" (Throat-God Temple).

EARLY MODERN PERIOD

The period from the fifteenth to the nineteenth century saw a dramatic rise in developments related to recognizing and attempting to treat esophageal cancer. The Spanish born Arabian physician Avenzoar (1090–1162), made several ingenious suggestions regarding cases of obstruction or of palsy of the gullet. He recommends treatment options that include "the introduction of food into the stomach by a silver tube and the use of nutritive enemata." However, Avenzoar did not recommend "support the strength by placing the patient in a tepid bath of nutritious liquids that might enter by cutaneous imbibition." One of the leading figures in sixteenth century science and medicine was the French born Jean Francois Fernel (1497–1558),[4] who wrote among other volumes, *On the Hidden Causes of Things* (1548) and *J. Fernelii Medicina* (1554) (**Fig. 4**). He described scirrhus and other tumors that blocked the esophagus, causing dysphagia.

In 1691, the surgeon John Casaubon died of esophageal cancer, and he described the symptoms leading up to his death.[5]

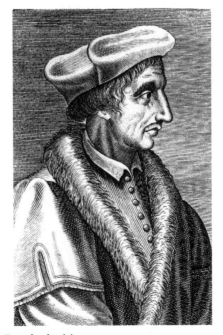

Fig. 4. Jean Fernel, the French physician.

At dinner I was almost choaked by swallowing a bit of a roasted mutton which as I thought stuck in the passage about the mouth of the stomach. But it suffered noething to goe downe and the stomach threw all up, though never soe small in quantitie, to all our amazements the sckilfull not knowing what 2 make of my condition. It being an unusuall afflixion wch. my melancholi suggested it an extra-ordinarie judgment. I could swallow about 2 spoonfulls about half way (as I thought) and then it would flush up in spite of my hart... Some small humidity or drops of what I dranck rather distilld or dropt into the stomach which afforded a bare living nourishment and on a sudden I grew lean as a skeleton and at some tymes very faint and feeble, although I recovered in some measure and had stomach 2 eate, my meate doeth noe gt. good and I am in a kind of atrophie...

From the commencement of the eighteenth century, reports of esophageal neoplasm were generally referred to as polypus, scirrhus, tumor, struma, or cartilaginous esophagus, and their description as either single case reports or case series was on the rise.

The first Western description suggesting a link with a history of heavy drinking and the development of esophageal cancer was made by E.G. Gyser in his 1770 paper titled, "*De fame lethali ex callosa oesophagi angustia.*"

The earliest drawings believed in existence of an esophageal neoplasm were published in Matthew Baillie's (**Fig. 5**)[6] 1799 edition of *Morbid Anatomy* (**Figs. 6–8**). In another book by Alexander T. Monro (1773–1859)[7] titled *The Morbid Anatomy of the Human Gullet, Stomach and Intestines*, published in 1881, Monro wrote about the treatment of "Scirrhus and cancer in the Gullet." Moreover, he mentioned the possibility of fatal esophagotracheal communication and was almost certainly the first

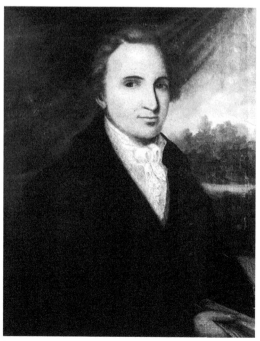

Fig. 5. Matthew Baillie.

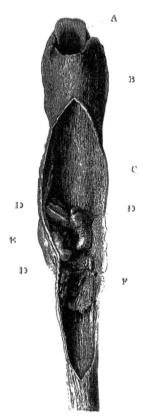

Fig. 6. "The same plate too represents some tumors in the cavity of the esophagus, forming a cause of obstruction in that canal which is very uncommon. … It is chiefly intended to represent three hard tumors which had grown from the inner surface of the esophagus, and which must have necessarily impeded very much deglutition. A: The epiglottis. B: The posterior surface of the pharynx. C: The esophagus laid open through nearly the whole of its extent. D: The three tumors which were growing from its extent. E: A lateral projection, or bulging of a part of the esophagus, occasioned by the growth of one of these tumors. F: An ulcerated surface, near which the parietes of the esophagus are a little thickened." (Baillie M. Series of engravings accompanied with explanations, which are intended to illustrate the morbid anatomy of some of the most important parts of the human body. London, Bulmer & Co. Plate II, Fig. II. 1799. p. 48–50.)

to describe the topic of the spread of "Scirrhus and Cancer" to and from the gullet. Furthermore, he describes the main symptoms plainly:[7]

> *Pain and an inability to swallow solids, are the earlier symptoms of this disease, and after a time, even fluids are arrested in their course downwards; they remain for a short time in the Gullet, and distend it, thereby creating a sense of suffocation, until the contents are rejected, by an inverted action of the Gullet, through the nose and mouth, by which the patient is much relieved, and the remainder passes down with a guggling noise, like water flowing through a constricted passage.*

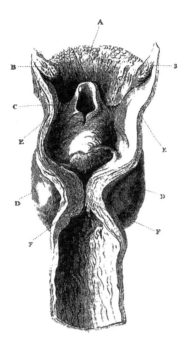

Fig. 7. "There is also sometimes a hard thickening of a part of the esophagus without ulcer, which may be considered as analogous to scirrhus in glandular parts. A: The upper surface of the posterior part of the tongue, which is crowded with follicles. B: The two tonsils. C: The epiglottis, with the aperture into the larynx. D: The posterior surface of the sides of the thyroid gland, which is a little enlarged. E: The cut edges of the pharynx, which is laid open. F: An ulcer at the upper extremity of the esophagus, with the sides a good deal thickened: the stricture therefore in this case was considerable. G: A part of the esophagus under an ulcer, where the structure is sound." (Baillie M. Series of engravings accompanied with explanations, which are intended to illustrate the morbid anatomy of some of the most important parts of the human body. London, Bulmer & Co. Plate III, Fig. II. 1799. p. 51–2.)

In 1825, a physician named John Howship (1781–1841)[8] was the author of *Practical Remarks upon Indigestion*, in which he made some important observations about esophageal tumors:

The oesophagus is occasionally subject to schirrus, or true cancer… All parts of the oesophagus are liable to this disease; and generally speaking, difficulty in swallowing, as in the early stages of other kinds of stricture, is here also among the earliest symptoms… But, of all diagnostic symptoms, sensations of shooting, heat, and burning in the part itself, more especially if the patient emaciates rapidly, seem to afford the most decisive evidence of the existence of schirrus, or cancer. Although, however, this sense of heat, if present, may clear up doubt, its absence must not remove suspicion; for of the two cases of this disease selected from those I have seen, in one there was a constant sense of intense burning heat in the part, compared to that of a red-hot poker boring through the back (Case 11); in the other, no feeling whatever, from first to last, of local pain was perceived, much less of those peculiar sensations generally attendant upon this disease, although after death it was found to possess every appearance of tuberculated schirrus (Case 10).

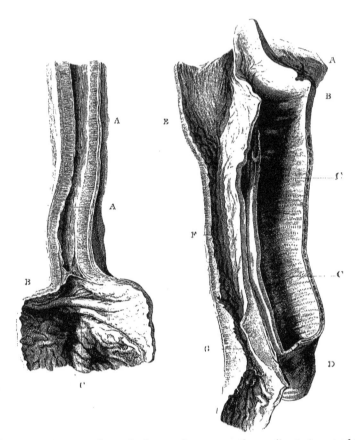

Fig. 8. "Fig. I. Represents a stricture in the esophagus near the cardia. A: A part of the boy of the os uoides, covered from view by the muscules which are attached to it. B: A lateral view of the cavity of the larynx. C: A lateral view of the cavity of the trachea. D: A part of the left bronchia. E: A lateral view of the cavity of the pharynx. F: A lateral view of the cavity of the esophagus in a sound state. G: A stricture near the cardia, where the sides of the esophagus are very thick and hard, and where there is some degree of ulceration upon the internal surface." "Fig. II. Represents a stricture in the esophagus of great extent, not attended with ulceration. The coats of the esophagus are very hard and much thickened, and upon the cut surface may be observed many white transverse lines. These represent the cellular membrane interposed between the muscular fibers, thickened from disease. This preparation may be considered as affording a good example of scirrhus in muscular parts. A: A considerable portion of the esophagus contracted in its cavity, and thickened in its substance. B: Shewing the canal to be very narrow at the cardia. C: A small part of the inner surface of the stomach, near the cardia, sound in its structure, and exhibiting some rugae." (Baillie M. Series of engravings accompanied with explanations, which are intended to illustrate the morbid anatomy of some of the most important parts of the human body. London, Bulmer & Co. Plate IV, Fig. I and II.1799. p. 53–4.)

Later, Howship mentioned that the dysphagia experienced in Case 10 was the result of spasmodic stricture of the upper esophagus induced by pathology at the cardia. In addition, Howship was believed to also be one of the first from the Western world to report that esophageal cancer rarely develops in early life.

There were several advances during this time, but none more important that the development of the esophagoscope. Adolf Kussmaul (1822–1902) **(Fig. 9)**[9] introduced this revolutionary device in 1868 when he passed a lighted tube through the entire esophagus into the stomach of a patient.

In terms of surgical advances, important esophageal resection and reanastomosis surgery conducted on animals (dogs)[10] in 1871 by Theodor Billroth (1829–1894) **(Fig. 10)** paved the way for surgical techniques in human beings. Billroth suggested that it was reasonable to resect a cervical esophageal cancer in humans. Then in 1877, Adolph Kussmaul's son-in-law, Vincenz Czerny (1842–1916) **(Fig. 11)**,[11] performed the first successful human resection of the cervical esophagus, after conducting animal experiments where he had resected a carcinoma of the cervical esophagus that provided a 1-year survival. However, perhaps one of Czerny's greatest proposals was that surgery alone would not be adequate for controlling cancer, leading to his development of concepts for multimodality treatment.[12] Then, in 1846, the publication of *The Nature and Treatment of Cancer* by W.H. Walshe (1812–1892) included the most substantial writings on esophageal cancer yet published. This publication included all aspects of the disease, including its incidence, site, form, type, metastases, symptoms, spread, differential diagnosis, and treatment. From his own clinical observations, Walshe concluded that cauterization of the cancerous obstruction of the esophagus lessened dysphagia and that in some cases "leeching the throat" had produced a good effect. At this time the only practical surgical option for esophageal cancer was esophagostomy.

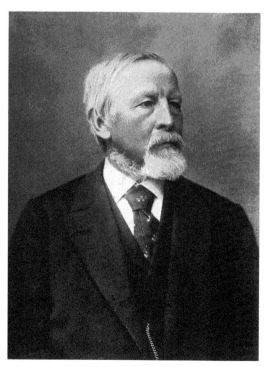

Fig. 9. Adolf Kussmaul, developer of the esophagoscope in 1868.

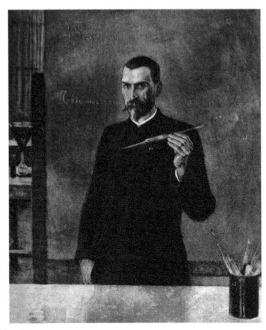

Fig. 10. Theodor Billroth.

MODERN ERA

The last 100 years have brought about a number of major developments in the diagnosis and treatment of esophageal cancer. This includes the development and refinement of surgical techniques, identification of Barrett's esophagus as a precursor to the development of esophageal cancer, improvements in endoscopy (ie, photography, magnification endoscopy, chromoendoscopy, capsule or wireless endoscopy, optical coherence endoscopy, light-induced fluorescence spectroscopy, endoscopic ultrasonography), radiology (computed tomography, MRI, positron emission tomography), and therapy (photodynamic therapy, argon plasma coagulation, thermal lasers, chemotherapy, radiation therapy).

At the commencement twentieth century there were numerous efforts around the world to treat esophageal cancer. There were several early successful attempts at esophageal resection and esophagectomy between 1909 and 1938 by surgeons in Germany,[13] Japan (Oshawa),[14] the United Kingdom (Evans, Lewis, Belsey),[15,16] and the United States (Torek, Adams, Phemister).[17–21]

A major pioneer in esophageal surgery was the Welsh surgeon, Ivor Lewis (1895–1982),[15] who in 1946 made substantial advancements with the introduction of esophagectomy and esophagogastrostomy through right-sided thoracotomy to prevent the problems associated with a left thoracotomy. The surgical experiences of World War II lay the foundations for new developments in esophageal surgery.

Another internationally renowned surgeon from the United Kingdom was Ronald H. Belsey (1910–2007), who developed the "Belsey Mark IV" operation for reflux in 1952. Moreover, he was also involved in the development of using the isoperistaltic left colon for replacement of the total esophagus. Because of the very poor

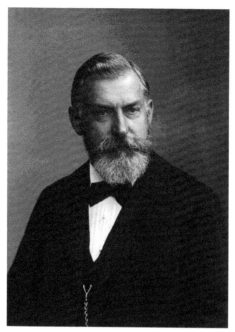

Fig. 11. Vincenz Czerny.

prognosis for esophageal cancer patients, Belsey once said "that the main goal was good palliation and that cure is an accident."[22]

Across the Atlantic in the United States, surgeon Franz Torek[21] performed the first transthoracic excision of a midesophageal carcinoma in 1913. The patient, a 67-year-old female, survived an additional 13 years in good health. In 1929, the Japanese surgeon Tohru Ohsawa[23] performed the world's first successful intrthoracic esophagojejunostomy with total gastrectomy. Moreover, in 1933, he undertook a series of transthoracic resections of the thoracic esophagus in 18 patients, with 8 patients surviving.

Surgery has normally been considered as "the only option" for patients with early stage cancer of the esophagus, and it wasn't until the mid-1980s that other combined therapy options became available to patients.[24] These combinations of therapies, known as "multimodality therapy," involve radiation, chemotherapy, or both before surgery for treatment of esophageal cancer. Unfortunately, even with these combined treatment options, the impact in terms of increased survival has not been impressive.

There are many other significant events in the history of esophageal cancer that one could write about, such as imaging, epidemiology, staging, and therapy options; however, surgery has been the main focus in terms of treatment options for esophageal cancer since the discovery of this lesion in the gullet in ancient times.

It is interesting to look back in time and see what developments have taken place and who the key people involved in making these events historic were. As one can see, there are many who have paved the way with the intent of "curing" this terrible disease, and each has played an important role in making this dream become a hopeful reality sometime in the twenty-first century.

ACKNOWLEDGMENTS

The author would like to thank the Center for the History of Medicine at the Countway Library of Medicine, Harvard Medical School, for assistance in finding reference sources and providing images, as well as the Wellcome Library for providing some of the images used in this article.

REFERENCES

1. Breasted JH. The Edwin Smith surgical papyrus: facsimile plates and line for line hieroglyphic transliteration. Whitefish, MT: Kessinger Publishing; 2006.
2. Brewer LA. History of surgery of the esophagus. Am J Surg 1980;139:730–43.
3. Qian ZX. Investigation on esophageal cancer in the province of Xinjiang. Collected papers of the second symposium on esophageal carcinoma. Chinese Acad Med Sci 1961:74–8.
4. Fernel J. (Leyden edition of 1645): De Morbis Universalibus et Particularibus. Lugduni Batavorum [Latin].
5. Casaubon J. Last entry in his diary, dated Monday 29 December, 1690, in catalogue of an exhibition of medical records. London: British Records Association; 1958. p. 30.
6. Baillie M. Series of engravings accompanied with explanations, which are intended to illustrate the morbid anatomy of some of the most important parts of the human body. London: Bulmer & Co.; 1799. p. 48–54.
7. Monro A. The morbid anatomy of the human gullet, stomach and intestines. London: Longman; 1881. p. 325.
8. Howship J. Practical remarks upon indigestion. London: Longman; 1825;22:161.
9. Kussmaul A. Zur geschicle der oesophago und gastroskopie. Arch Klin Med 1898;6:456 [German].
10. Billroth T. Ueber die resection des oesophagus. Arch Klin Chir 1871;13:65–9 [German].
11. Czerny V. Neue operationen. Zentralbl Chir 1877;4:433–4 [German].
12. Willeke F, Lehnert T. Vincenz Czerny: carrying concepts into the 21st century. Eur J Surg Oncol 1997;23:253–6.
13. Denk W. Zur radikaloperation des oesophaguskarzinoms. Zentralbl Chir 1913;40: 1065 [German].
14. Imamura M, Tobe T. Intrathoracic esophagojejunostomy following the resection of the lower esophagus—Tohru Ohsawa, pioneer in surgery of the esophagus. World J Surg 1985;9:645–7.
15. Lewis I. The surgical treatment of carcinoma of the oesophagus with special reference to the new operation for growths in the middle third. Br J Surg 1946;34: 18–31.
16. Morris-Stiff G, Hughes LE. Ivor Lewis (1895–1982) Welsh pioneer of the right-sided approach to the oesophagus. Dig Surg 2003;20:546–53.
17. Adams WE, Phemister DB. Carcinoma of the lower thoracic esophagus: report of a successful resection and esophagogastrectomy. J Thorac Surg 1938;7:62.
18. Klingman RR, DeMeester TR. Surgery for carcinoma of the thoracic esophagus: Adams and Phemister in perspective. Ann Thorac Surg 1988;46:699–702.
19. Dubecz A, Schwartz SI. Franz John A. Torek. Ann Thorac Surg 2008;85:1497–9.
20. Naef AP. William E. Adams: Thomas Mann and the magic mountain. Ann Thorac Surg 1998;65:285–7.
21. Torek F. The first successful case of resection of the thoracic portion of the oesophagus for carcinoma. Surg Gynecol Obstet 1913;16:614.

22. Lerut T. Esophageal surgery at the end of the millennium. J Thorac Cardiovasc Surg 1998;116:1–20.
23. Ohsawa T. The surgery of the oesophagus. J Chir 1933;10:604.
24. Leichman L. Preoperative chemotherapy and radiation therapy for patients with cancer of the esophagus: a potentially curative approach. J Clin Oncol 1984;2: 75–9.

Epidemiology of Esophageal Cancer

Guy D. Eslick, PhD, MMedSc (Clin Epi), MMedStat*

KEYWORDS

• Epidemiology • Incidence • Esophageal • Cancer • Mortality

The epidemiology of esophageal cancer is fascinating, yet remains very poorly understood. Advances in data collection and surveillance, not to mention the development of national cancer registries to collect incidence data in developed and developing countries, have provided more accurate monitoring of this disease over the last few decades. Currently, esophageal cancer is the eighth most common incident cancer in the world and, because of its extremely aggressive nature and poor survival rate, it ranks sixth among all cancers in mortality.[1,2] Despite these facts, esophageal cancer receives very little mention when compared with other cancers such as lung, breast, and colon in terms of health promotion and education. Special note, however, should be given to the fact that esophageal cancer is one of the very few cancers that is contributing to increasing death rates (20%) among males in the United States.[3] Understanding and delineating the epidemiology of esophageal cancer will be the key to elucidating the causes and risk factors for esophageal cancer and thus the cornerstone of developing any prevention strategies.

EPIDEMIOLOGY
Age

The incidence of esophageal cancer increases with age. This pattern is similar in developing and developed countries. On average, adenocarcinoma generally is acquired 10 years earlier than squamous cell carcinoma (**Table 1**).

Gender

In terms of gender differences, for squamous cell carcinoma in the Western world it occurs three to four times more often in males than females, although in the esophageal cancer belt, it is approximately a one to one ratio. for adenocarcinoma, however,

The author's work is supported by The International Union Against Cancer and the American Cancer Society (ACS) with an International Fellowship for Beginning Investigators (ACSBI).

School of Public Health, The University of Sydney, Sydney, New South Wales, Australia

* Corresponding author. Program in Molecular and Genetic Epidemiology Harvard School of Public Health, 677 Huntington Avenue, Building II, 2nd Floor, Room. 209, Boston, MA 02115.

E-mail address: geslick@hsph.harvard.edu

Gastroenterol Clin N Am 38 (2009) 17–25

doi:10.1016/j.gtc.2009.01.008

gastro.theclinics.com

Table 1
Comparison of squamous cell carcinoma and adenocarcinoma of the esophagus

	Squamous Cell Carcinoma	Adenocarcinoma
Age	60–70 years; median 62.7 years	50–60 years; median 53.4 years
Gender	Male	Male
Socioeconomic status	Low	Middle to upper
Locations	75% midesophagus	94% distal esophagus
Symptoms	Progressive dysphagia, odynophagia, halitosis, unintentional weight loss, chest pain	Progressive dysphagia, odynophagia, halitosis, unintentional weight loss, chest pain
Environmental factors	Alcohol, cigarette smoking, mate-tea ingestion, betel-nut chewing, caustic ingestion, esophageal radiation exposure, high-fat diet, low vitamin diet [vitamin C, folate, beta-carotene, vitamin E], drinking hot liquids (>70°C)	Cigarette smoking, high-fat diet, low vitamin diet [vitamin C, folate, beta-carotene, vitamin E]
Medical conditions	Head/neck squamous cell carcinoma, Plummer-Vinson [Patterson-Kelly] syndrome, achalasia, tylosis, celiac disease, human papilloma virus infection, *Helicobacter pylori* infection	Barrett's metaplasia, Zollinger-Ellison syndrome, scleroderma, prior esophageal dilations, gastroesophageal reflux disease, obesity

males are six to eight times more likely to develop this particular form of esophageal cancer than females.[4]

World

Esophageal cancer is an uncommon cancer. In terms of new (incident) cases of cancer, esophageal cancer is ranked as the eighth most common cancer in the world. At this point, it is important to differentiate esophageal cancer into its two histopathological subtypes (squamous cell carcinoma and adenocarcinoma), as the epidemiology between the two groups is vastly different. Surprisingly, over the last 30 years, there has been a major shift in the dominating histologic subtype of esophageal cancer in the Western world; previously, it was squamous cell carcinoma, and now it is adenocarcinoma.[4] It is important to note that the classification of esophago–cardial adenocarcinomas also may explain the increase in this lesion. The wide geographic variation in incidence of esophageal cancer is marked, as is the mortality rates (**Fig. 1**). The variation in incidence for esophageal cancer can differ as much as 500-fold from one part of the world to another. It is known that Asian countries, in particular China, India, Pakistan, and Japan, have the highest rates of esophageal cancer in the world; therefore countries mentioned in the following sections highlight those that have changed substantially over time or those that may not be well known as having high incidence of esophageal cancer.

United States

It is surprising to find that in the United States the incidence of esophageal cancer among both males and females ranks in the top 20 countries. Disturbingly, African American males from the District of Columbia rank number five and African American females from the state of Connecticut rank number 14 (**Tables 2** and **3**). Moreover, African Americans from two additional states (South Carolina and Georgia) also are listed in the top 20 locations for esophageal cancer in the world. In the United States, squamous cell carcinoma remains the predominant subtype among African Americans, who have esophageal cancer rates six times higher than whites.[4–7]

The latest cancer statistics estimated that 16,470 new (incident) cases of esophageal cancer were expected to occur in the United States in 2008.[3] This included an estimated 12,970 males and 3500 females. An expected 14,280 deaths from esophageal cancer (11,250 male and 3,030 female) also were estimated. This makes esophageal cancer the seventh highest among males in estimated deaths from all cancer sites, which represents 4%.

In terms of the total contribution of esophageal cancer to the decrease in cancer death rates, females showed a small decrease (0.4%) in cancer deaths between 1990 and 2004. However, for males there has been no such decrease, in fact there has been staggering astounding 19.7% increase.[3]

Survival rates between 1996 and 2003 by ethnicity also reveal differences. Although generally the distribution of esophageal cancer (localized, regional, distant) shows no real differences at diagnosis, the 5-year survival rates (%) between whites and African Americans appears significant, with localized lesions (36% versus 20%) and regional lesions (18% versus 11%) showing the greatest differences. For distant lesions (3% versus 2%), however, there is no difference in survival rates. Trends over time of survival rates between African Americans and whites have changed slightly; 5-year survival rates from 1975 to 1977 were 6%, 3%, and 5% for whites, African Americans, and all races. From 1984 to 1986 they were 11%, 8%, and 10%, and from 1996 to 1998, they were 18%, 11% and 16%, respectively.[3]

United Kingdom

In terms of world rank, esophageal cancer incidence rates in the United Kingdom are fairly high, and this appears to be greater for females than males as Scotland, Merseyside and Cheshire, West Midlands, Trent, South and Western, Northern and Yorkshire, and Ireland are all ranked in the top 20 locations for esophageal cancer for females, while only Scotland (ranked 17) appears for the males (see **Tables 2** and **3**).

A recent study examined the national incidence rates of esophageal adenocarcinoma in England and Wales between 1971 and 2001 using the largest population-based cancer registry.[8] There were a total of 43,753 cases of esophageal adenocarcinoma over the 31-year period. The age standardized world incidence rates increased rapidly by 39.6% (95% CI: 38.6 to 40.6) and 37.5% (95% CI: 35.8-39.2), for males and females, respectively. This dramatic increase in esophageal adenocarcinoma was especially prominent among those aged 50 to 54 years in both males and females. Increases in incidence occurred across all socioeconomic levels; however, those in the more affluent groups had a higher incidence of esophageal adenocarcinoma compared with all other groups, including the most deprived. Based on these data, the authors suggest that for those born in 1940 or later, that esophageal adenocarcinoma will soon cease being a rare cancer.[8]

An earlier study reported the incidence rates for esophageal cancer in the United Kingdom, which included Scotland, England-Wales, Northern Ireland, France,

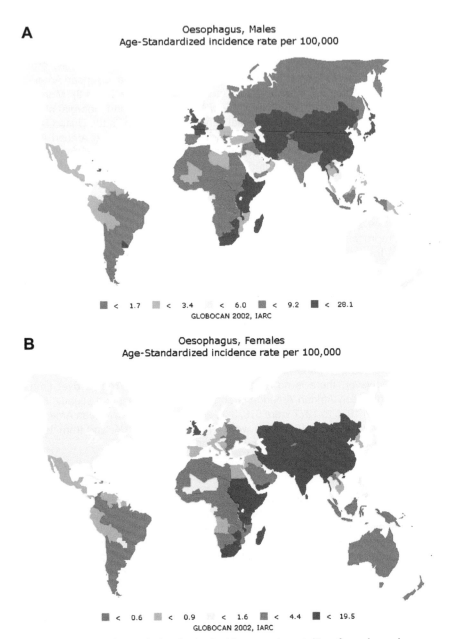

A

Oesophagus, Males
Age-Standardized incidence rate per 100,000

■ < 1.7 ■ < 3.4 < 6.0 ■ < 9.2 ■ < 28.1
GLOBOCAN 2002, IARC

B

Oesophagus, Females
Age-Standardized incidence rate per 100,000

■ < 0.6 ■ < 0.9 < 1.6 ■ < 4.4 ■ < 19.5
GLOBOCAN 2002, IARC

Fig. 1. (A–D) Geographic variation in the incidence and mortality of esophageal cancer.

Portugal, Spain, Germany, Belgium, Italy, Denmark, Netherlands, and Greece for the periods 1960 to 1964 to 1985 to1989.[9] They found that esophageal cancer rates had been increasing during the 40-year period among both males and females in the United Kingdom, and that squamous cell carcinoma had been overtaken by adenocarcinoma as the leading histologic subtype; this was also reported in a separate study from Finland.[10] France consistently had produced the highest incidence rates for

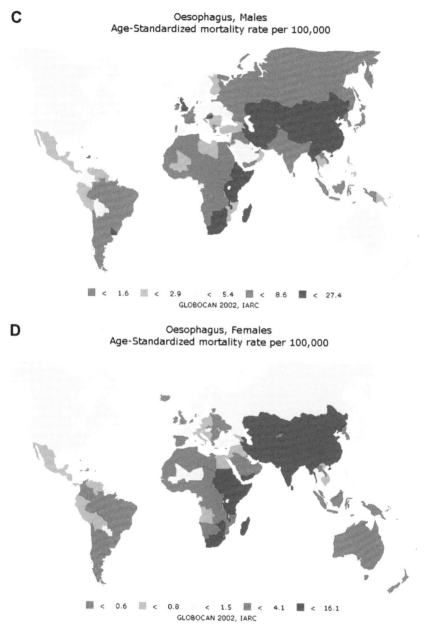

C

Oesophagus, Males
Age-Standardized mortality rate per 100,000

< 1.6   < 2.9   < 5.4   < 8.6   < 27.4
GLOBOCAN 2002, IARC

D

Oesophagus, Females
Age-Standardized mortality rate per 100,000

< 0.6   < 0.8   < 1.5   < 4.1   < 16.1
GLOBOCAN 2002, IARC

Fig. 1. (*continued*).

males (see **Table 3**), while Greece had the lowest rates. Other European countries including Denmark, Netherlands, and Spain also showed significant increases in the number of new cases of esophageal cancer. In addition, mortality data from 1911 to 1986 to 1989 for Scotland, England, and Wales comparing males and females showed that in general for all locations and for both genders that mortality rates were

Table 2
World age standard rates (per 100,000 population) for males with esophageal cancer (GLOBOCAN 2002, International Agency for Research on Cancer)

Country, State/Province	Cases	Age Standard Rate
1. China, Jiashan	254	20.2
2. China, Zhongshan	532	16.5
3. Japan, Miyagi	1656	15.4
4. Zimbabwe, Harare: African	219	15.1
5. USA, District of Columbia: black	149	14.8
6. France, Calvados	327	14.6
7. United States, South Carolina: black	377	14.4
8. France, Somme	271	14.1
9. Uganda, Kyadondo	125	14.1
10. France, Manche	268	13.1
11. Brazil, Brasilia	262	13.1
12. Japan, Yamagata	892	13.0
13. France, Loire-Atlantique	503	12.7
14. Japan, Hiroshima	503	12.1
15. Brazil, Sao Paulo	2406	12.0
16. Brazil, Cuiaba	72	11.7
17. United Kingdom, Scotland	2391	11.7
18. United States, Georgia: Black	470	11.1
19. France, Bas-Rhin	370	10.9
20. United States, District of Columbia	179	10.8

increasing. Mortality rates for males in England and Wales, however, were higher between 1911 and 1931; then they dropped until 1955, at which point they started increasing rapidly to similar rates reported in 1911.[9]

Africa

There are very limited data from African countries in terms of cancer incidence and mortality rates. A study in Kenya that aimed to determine rates of esophageal cancer in the North Rift Valley by reviewing all pathology records between 1994 and 2001 from a teaching and referral hospital, however, found that esophageal cancer was the most common cancer in males and the third most common among females.[11] There was no real gender difference with the male to female ratio being 1.5:1; however, certain geographic locations had higher rates for females compared with males. The mean age of patients was 59 years, and squamous cell carcinoma accounted for 90% of the lesions. It is of note that Zimbabwe has the highest incidence of esophageal cancer for both males and females (see **Tables 2 and 3**), ranked fourth among males and fifth among females.

Thailand

There is very little in the literature on esophageal cancer rates in Thailand. One study reviewed records of provincial hospitals of Haadyai, Yala, Pattani, Satun, and Nartiwat

Table 3
World age standard rates (per 100,000 population) for females with esophageal cancer (GLOBOCAN 2002, International Agency for Research on Cancer)

Country, State/Province	Cases	Age Standard Rate
1. Pakistan, South Karachi	166	8.6
2. Uganda, Kyadondo	78	8.4
3. India, Nagpur	214	5.7
4. India, Chennai	479	5.4
5. Zimbabwe, Harare: African	67	5.3
6. India, Poona	295	5.0
7. Chile, Valdivia	51	4.9
8. China, Jiashan	70	4.8
9. United Kingdom, Scotland	1524	4.7
10. India, Mumbai	905	4.6
11. United Kingdom, Merseyside and Cheshire	692	4.6
12. United Kingdom, West Midlands	1347	4.1
13. Brazil, Brasilia	95	3.9
14. United States, Connecticut: black	36	3.9
15. United Kingdom, North Western	992	3.8
16. United Kingdom, Trent	1176	3.8
17. India, New Delhi	598	3.6
18. United Kingdom, South and Western	1792	3.6
19. United Kingdom, Northern and Yorkshire	1525	3.6
20. Ireland	597	3.5

between 1981 and 1983.[12] Esophageal cancer was the leading cancer for males (18%) and ranked fourth among females (5.73%); dysphagia was present in 90% of cases, with a wide duration ranging between 5 days and 6 months. All cases were squamous cell carcinoma, and most lesions were found in the middle third of the esophagus

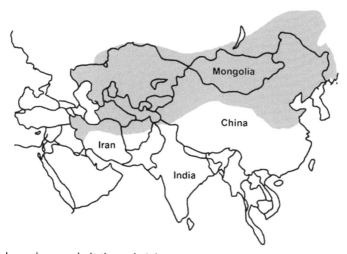

Fig. 2. Esophageal cancer belt through Asia.

(53%). Twenty-seven percent were found in the upper third, and 20% were reported in the lower third of the esophagus. All patients died within 6 months.

Asian Esophageal Cancer Belt

It is important to briefly mention the esophageal cancer belt (**Fig. 2**), which passes from Turkey through countries such as Iraq, Iran, and Kazakhstan, and on to Northern China. Most esophageal cancers in this region are squamous cell carcinomas. This region has the highest incidence rates for esophageal cancer in the world. Assessment of these differences, not only between countries, but more importantly within countries, where there may be a 500-fold difference between two locations 100 miles apart, is being undertaken using spatial analysis.[13–15]

SUMMARY

There is no doubt that the epidemiology of esophageal cancer has changed substantially over the last 50 years, especially in the Western World, with the traditionally dominant squamous cell carcinoma being overtaken by adenocarcinoma. The incidence is increasing at very rapid rates for both males and females, and this has caused a shift in the epidemiology of esophageal cancer, which is now more likely to affect more affluent white men. Esophageal cancer has increased more rapidly than any other cancer in the Western world. The reasons for this striking increase remain largely unexplained. Esophageal cancer always has been a major public health issue in countries with traditionally high incidence such as China, and with dramatic changes in Western countries such as the United States, the impetus must be directed at finding answers for these changes in epidemiology, which in turn should provide insight into etiologic factors and lead to primary prevention of this devastating disease.

REFERENCES

1. Parkin DM, Bray F, Ferlay J, et al. Global Cancer Statistics, 2002. CA Cancer J Clin 2005;55:74–108.
2. Kamangar F, Dores GM, Anderson WF. Patterns of cancer incidence, mortality, and prevalence across five continents: defining priorities to reduce cancer disparities in different geographic regions of the world. J Clin Oncol 2006;24:2137–50.
3. Jemal A, Siegel R, Ward E, et al. Cancer statistics, 2008. CA Cancer J Clin 2008;58:71–96.
4. Blot WJ, Devesa SS, Kneller RW, et al. Rising incidence of adenocarcinoma of the esophagus and gastric cardia. JAMA 1991;265:1287–9.
5. Greenstein AJ, Litle VR, Swanson SJ, et al. Racial disparities in esophageal cancer treatment and outcomes. Ann Surg Oncol 2008;15:881–8.
6. Trivers KF, Sabatino SA, Stewart SL. Trends in esophageal cancer incidence by histology, United Stats, 1998–2003. Int J Cancer 2008;123:1422–8.
7. Baquet CR, Commiskey P, Mack S, et al. Esophageal cancer epidemiology in blacks and whites: racial and gender disparities in incidence, mortality, survival rates and histology. J Natl Med Assoc 2005;97:1471–8.
8. Lapage C, Rachet B, Jooste V, et al. Continuing rapid increase in esophageal adenocarcinoma in England and Wales. Am J Gastroenterol 2008;103:2694–9.
9. Macfarlane GJ, Boyle P. The epidemiology of oesophageal cancer in the UK and other European countries. J R Soc Med 1994;87:334–7.

10. Voutilainen ME, Juhola MT. The changing epidemiology of esophageal cancer in Finland and the impact of the surveillance of Barrett's esophagus in detecting esophageal adenocarcinoma. Dis Esophagus 2005;18:221–5.
11. Wakhisi J, Patel K, Buziba N, et al. Esophageal cancer in north rift valley of western Kenya. Afr Health Sci 2005;5:156–63.
12. Chanvithan A, Ubolcholket S. Carcinoma of the esophagus in Muslims of Southern Thailand: epidemiology. Thailand Journal of Surgery 1984;5:113–6.
13. Bader F, Anwar N, Mahmood S. Geographical variation in the epidemiology of esophageal cancer in Pakistan. Asian Pac J Cancer Prev 2005;6:139–42.
14. Mohebbi M, Mahmoodi M, Wolfe R, et al. Geographical spread of gastrointestinal tract cancer incidence in the Caspian Sea region of Iran: spatial analysis of cancer registry data. BMC Cancer 2008;8:137.
15. Wu KS, Huo X, Zhu GH. Relationships between esophageal cancer and spatial environment factors by using geographic information systems. Sci Total Environ 2008;393:219–25.

Environmental Causes of Esophageal Cancer

Farin Kamangar, MD, PhD[a],*, Wong-Ho Chow, PhD[b],
Christian C. Abnet, PhD, MPH[c], Sanford M. Dawsey, MD[d]

KEYWORDS

- Esophageal cancer • Risk factor • Tobacco
- Alcohol • Socioeconomic status • Obesity
- Acid reflux • Helicobacter pylori

Esophageal cancer (EC) is the eighth most common incident cancer in the world and, because of its high fatality rate, ranks sixth among all cancers in mortality.[1,2] It is not surprising, therefore, that the etiology of EC has been investigated for over a century. Based on clinical observations, Craver[3] in 1932 and Watson[4] in 1939 listed excessive use of alcohol and tobacco, low socioeconomic status, poor oral health, and consumption of hot drinks as risk factors for EC. They also cited papers on EC etiology published decades earlier. For example, Craver cites a 1920 article from Argentina that suggests maté drinking as a risk factor for EC.

Etiology of EC differs by histology. EC can be histologically classified into two main types: esophageal squamous cell carcinoma (ESCC) and esophageal adenocarcinoma (EA). These cancer types differ not only histologically, but also with respect to their incidence trends, populations that they affect, and risk factors. One could call EA an emerging disease. Until the 1970s, ESCC constituted the large majority (over 90%) of all EC cases in all parts of the world. Since then, incidence rates of EA have sharply increased in many countries in the Western world,[5–9] so that this cancer type now constitutes approximately half of all EC cases in some Western countries. In contrast, ESCC continues to be the dominant type in the rest of the world.

Most etiologic studies conducted before the 1980s did not distinguish between ESCC and EA, but their results were mainly relevant to ESCC, because EA was

Writing this review article was supported by the Intramural Research Program of the National Cancer Institute, National Institutes of Health.

[a] Division of Cancer Epidemiology and Genetics, NCI, 6120 Executive Blvd., Room 3034, Bethesda, MD 20892-7232, USA
[b] Division of Cancer Epidemiology and Genetics, NCI, 6120 Executive Blvd., Room 8100, Bethesda, MD 20892-7240, USA
[c] Division of Cancer Epidemiology and Genetics, NCI, 6120 Executive Blvd., Room 3042, Bethesda, MD 20892-7232, USA
[d] Division of Cancer Epidemiology and Genetics, NCI, 6120 Executive Blvd., Room 3024, Bethesda, MD 20892-7232, USA
* Corresponding author.
E-mail address: kamangaf@mail.nih.gov (F. Kamangar).

uncommon before then. Also, results of the more recent studies from Asia, South America, or Africa that do not report histology are mainly applicable to ESCC because EA is still relatively uncommon in these areas.[10–12] Extensive investigations into the etiology of EA started in the 1990s, mainly in Western countries, where larger numbers of this cancer began to be diagnosed.

Some parts of the world have distinct epidemiologic patterns of ESCC. In most parts of the world, incidence rates of ESCC, adjusted to the 1970 world population, are lower than 15 per 10^5 person-years and ESCC is two to three times more common in men than in women.[13] However, in certain areas of China (in the Taihang mountain region) and Iran (in Golestan Province), a completely different pattern is observed: incidence rates above 100 per 10^5 person-years have been reported, and men and women have similar incidence rates.[13] ESCC risk factors in these areas may be different from those seen elsewhere. For example, unlike almost everywhere else, tobacco smoking and alcohol consumption play a minor role.[14,15]

ESCC and EA have known precursor lesions, esophageal squamous dysplasia (ESD) and Barrett esophagus (BE), respectively. Compared with subjects with no ESD, those with mild, moderate, and severe ESD have an increased risk of ESCC of approximately 3-, 10-, and 30-fold, respectively.[16] Presence of BE substantially increases EA risk; risk of progression to EA is 0.5% to 1% per year.[17,18] Therefore, ESD and BE have been used as surrogate endpoints for ESCC and EA, respectively.

With this background, the authors review some factors that increase or decrease EC risk. Where data are available, the effect of each factor separately for ESCC and EA is discussed. Many factors have been investigated in relation to EC. Within these, the authors have chosen those that are established risk factors, or those for which there is substantial data, or those for which there is currently strong research interest. These factors include:

Habits—tobacco use, alcohol consumption, opium consumption, maté drinking, consumption of hot drinks, consumption of carbonated soft drinks, eating pickled vegetables

Nutritional deficiencies—low intake of fresh fruit and vegetables, vitamin and mineral deficiencies

Medications—nonsteroidal anti-inflammatory drugs (NSAIDs), medications that relax the lower esophageal sphincter (LES), histamine2 (H_2) receptor antagonists

Infections—*Helicobacter pylori*, human papillomavirus (HPV)

Chemical carcinogens—polycyclic aromatic hydrocarbons (PAH), nitrosamines, acetaldehyde

Physiologic or pathologic predisposing conditions—gastroesophageal acid reflux, hiatal hernia, achalasia, gastric atrophy, poor oral health

Occupational exposure—to silica and asbestos

Low socioeconomic status

Box 1 contains a more detailed outline.

HABITS
Tobacco Use

As early as 1979, the US Surgeon General[19] reported that, "Cigarette smoking is a significant causal factor in the development of EC. The risk … increases with the amount smoked." The 1989 Surgeon General report[20] added that: "The proportion of EC deaths attributable to tobacco use in the United States is estimated to be

78 percent for men and 75 percent for women." Since the publication of these reports, a large number of case-control and cohort studies have confirmed these statements.

Cigarette smoking is more strongly associated with ESCC than with EA. Studies have shown that ESCC risk is increased approximately three-fold to seven-fold in current smokers.[21–25] Smoking cigars or a pipe confers risks similar to cigarette smoking.[26] The International Agency for Research on Cancer (IARC) has concluded that chewing betel quid that includes tobacco, which is common in South and South-East Asia, can also cause ESCC.[27] There is less data available for other forms of tobacco use, such as using water pipe (hookah) and chewing nass (a mixture of lime, ash, and tobacco), which are predominantly used in the Middle-East. However, these forms of tobacco also seem to increase ESCC risk.[28] The only exceptions to a strong association with tobacco have been reported from the very high-risk regions of China (in the Taihang mountain region) and Iran (in Golestan Province). In these areas, cigarette smoking is a minor risk factor for ESCC, with relative risk of approximately 1.5.[12,28,29] It is unclear why the association is much weaker in these areas than what has been observed in the rest of the world. One hypothesis is that other strong risk factors may exist in these high-risk areas that account for the majority of the cases, and therefore the effect of smoking is diluted.[30]

Although smoking is less strongly associated with EA, there is now little doubt that smoking is a risk factor for EA. At least 10 population-based case-control studies[31–40] and a large-scale cohort study[25] have evaluated the association between cigarette smoking and EA, and almost all of these studies have found an increased risk of nearly two-fold. Several of these studies have also shown a dose-response relationship. The consistency of association and the dose-response relationship both indicate a causal relationship. Further supporting this causal relationship is the effect of smoking in causing cancers in other organs,[41,42] and the presence of a large number of carcinogens, such as polycyclic aromatic hydrocarbons, nitrosamines, and acetaldehyde in tobacco smoke.[43] Also, because smoking starts years before tumor formation, there is no doubt about the direction of temporal relationship. Indeed the 2004 report of the US Surgeon General on health consequences of smoking concluded that there is sufficient evidence for a causal relationship between cigarette smoking and EA.[26]

Alcohol Consumption

Like tobacco use, alcohol consumption has long been known to be a major cause of EC in most areas of the world. Classic ecologic and case-control studies by Tuyns and others[44–47] in the 1970s and 1980s established alcohol as a strong cause of EC in many countries, and showed that alcohol drinking and tobacco smoking interact to increase EC risk in a multiplicative manner. IARC has classified alcohol drinking as a known cause of EC.[48]

The increased risk of EC associated with alcohol use is perhaps limited to ESCC. When used in excessive amounts (three or more drinks per day), alcohol has almost universally been associated with an elevated risk of ESCC; it typically increases risk by three-fold to five-fold.[25,49–51] In contrast, there is little evidence for an association between alcohol drinking and EA. The majority of the case-control and cohort studies that have investigated this association have found no overall relationship between alcohol consumption and EA, or have found relatively weak associations, both direct and inverse.[25,31–33,35,36,38,39,52] Some studies have suggested that only certain types of alcohol may be associated with EA. For example, one study suggested that drinking straight liquor could increase risk[32] and another one suggested that drinking wine may reduce risk.[33] These results need to be confirmed in other studies.

Box 1
Environmental risk factors and predisposing conditions for esophageal cancer

Habits

Tobacco use

> There is strong evidence for a causal association between tobacco use and both ESCC and EA

> Tobacco use is more strongly associated with ESCC—three-fold to seven-fold increased risk, than EA—two-fold increased risk

Alcohol consumption

> Excessive alcohol use—greater than three drinks per day—is a strong risk factor for ESCC, increasing risk by three-fold to five-fold

> There is little evidence for an association between alcohol use and EA risk

Opium use

> Studies point toward an association with ESCC—two-fold increased risk, but the level of evidence is not yet strong

Drinking maté

> Epidemiologic studies have consistently shown an increased risk of EC associated with drinking maté, especially hot maté

> Most studies have been conducted in areas with high prevalence of ESCC

Ingestions of high-temperature foods and drinks

> A large number of epidemiologic studies have investigated the association of hot foods and drinks with EC, but the results are still controversial

Consumption of carbonated soft drinks

> Results from epidemiologic studies have shown no evidence for an increased risk of EA or ESCC associated with drinking carbonated soft drinks

Eating pickled vegetables

> Eating pickled vegetables was once considered an important risk factor for EC in China, but the results of epidemiologic studies have been controversial

Nutritional deficiencies

Low intake of fresh fruits and vegetables

> There is a large body of evidence linking low intake of fresh fruits and vegetables to higher risk of EC, especially ESCC

> Eating 50 additional grams of fruits and vegetables per day may decrease EC risk by 20%

Vitamin and micronutrient deficiency

> Most vitamins and minerals do not change EC risk. However, intake of selenium in selenium-deficient populations may decrease ESCC risk, especially in younger people

Medications

Nonsteroidal anti-inflammatory drugs (NSAIDs)

> There is evidence that intake of aspirin and other NSAIDs may decrease both ESCC and EA by approximately 40%

Medications that relax lower esophageal sphincter (LES)

> LES-relaxing drugs have been suggested to increase EA risk by increasing acid reflux. However, the results of epidemiologic studies have been controversial

H2 receptor antagonists

> Although some studies have shown an increased risk of EA associated with taking these drugs, these results may be confounded by inadequate adjustment for acid reflux

Infections

Helicobacter pylori

Presence of *H pylori* in the stomach is associated with a 50% reduced risk of EA

There is no clear pattern of association between *H pylori* and ESCC

Human papillomavirus (HPV)

A large number of epidemiologic studies have investigated the association of HPV with EC, but the results are still controversial

Chemical carcinogens

Polycyclic aromatic hydrocarbons (PAHs)

There is circumstantial evidence linking PAHs to EC, but there is no convincing evidence from case-control or cohort studies

N-nitroso compounds (NNCs)

Intake of processed meat, which contains large amounts of NNCs, has been consistently linked to higher EC risk, but more evidence is required to make a causal link between NNCs and EC

Acetaldehyde

Acetaldehyde may be the common denominator linking alcohol consumption, poor oral health, and gastric atrophy to EC

The most convincing evidence for an association between acetaldehyde and EC comes from alcohol dehydrogenase and acetaldehyde dehydrogenase polymorphism studies, but more evidence is needed to make a causal link

Fumonisins

Ecologic studies have linked fumonisin exposure to increased risk of EC, but additional individual-based epidemiologic studies are needed to establish or refute this association

Predisposing conditions

Gastroesophageal acid reflux

Acid reflux is one of the main risk factors for EA, increasing its risk by approximately five-fold

Obesity

There is strong evidence for a causal association between obesity and higher risk of EA

Hiatal hernia

Hiatal hernia increases EA risk by two-fold to six-fold, most likely by increasing gastroesophageal acid reflux

Achalasia

Achalasia increases the risk of both EA and ESCC by approximately 10-fold

Gastric atrophy

A few studies have shown that gastric atrophy could be a risk factor for ESCC but more studies are needed to confirm these results. There is no evidence for an association between gastric atrophy and EA

Poor oral health

Several epidemiologic studies have linked poor oral health to higher risk of EC, especially ESCC, but more evidence is required to conclude that there is a causal association

Others

Occupational exposure

A number of studies have linked occupational exposure to silica and asbestos to higher risk of EC, but the results have not been entirely consistent

Low socioeconomic status

Low socioeconomic status is a risk factor for EC. It is a definite risk factor for ESCC, but it may also increase risk of EA

The exact mechanism of carcinogenicity of alcohol is not known, because alcohol itself does not bind DNA, is not mutagenic, and does not cause cancer in animals.[52] However, several mechanisms for its carcinogenicity have been suggested, including its conversion to acetaldehyde (see later discussion), acting as a solvent for other carcinogens, and causing nutritional deficiency.[53]

Opium Use

A role for opium as a potential cause of EC was first suggested when ecologic studies showed very high rates of opium consumption in high-risk areas of northeastern Iran. In a study of 1,590 rural individuals, the prevalence of appreciable levels (≥ 1 μg/ml) of urinary morphine metabolites was almost six-fold higher among residents of high-risk versus low-risk areas.[54] This study also compared household members of 41 cases and 41 matched controls for urinary opium metabolites and found a nonsignificant two-fold increased risk among case household members.[54] The results of a recent case-control study in this same area also showed that opium use was associated with a two-fold increased risk of EC.[28]

Crude opium, itself, is not mutagenic in the Ames test.[55,56] However, smoking opium may produce polycyclic aromatic hydrocarbons or other carcinogenic compounds. Opium dross and smoke condensates from opium and morphine cause mutations in *Salmonella typhimurium*,[55,56] sister chromatid exchanges in human lymphocytes,[57] and morphologic transformations in cultured Syrian hamster embryo cells.[58]

Although the results of the studies conducted thus far suggest that opium use could increase EC risk, the level of evidence for this association is not yet strong enough to be convincing. Data from case-control studies may be subject to recall or observer biases, and associations found in these studies may be due to reverse causation. The results of an ongoing cohort study in northern Iran will provide further evidence to evaluate this potential association.[59]

Drinking Maté

Maté, an infusion of the herb *Ilex paraguayensis* (also known as yerba maté), is commonly consumed, sometimes in large volumes (1–2 L/d), in some areas of South America, including southern Brazil, northeastern Argentina, Uruguay, and Paraguay.[60,61] These areas also have the highest risks of EC that are seen in South America.[62] Therefore, several case-control studies in these countries have examined the association between drinking maté and EC, and nearly all have found an increased risk.[63–69] A combined analysis of five of these studies showed a dose-response association with amount, duration, and temperature of maté drinking, with a relative risk of three in those who drank over 3 L of maté per day.[61]

Two independent mechanisms may explain the carcinogenicity of maté: repeated thermal injury, resulting from drinking hot maté, and exposure to polycyclic aromatic hydrocarbons (PAHs) that are found in maté.[70] Maté is often consumed hot or very hot, but it also can be consumed warm or cold. In 1991, IARC classified hot maté as a probable (Group 2A) carcinogen to humans,[71] implying that repeated thermal injury was the probable mechanism of carcinogenicity. However, several studies have now suggested that contaminants, especially PAHs, may also be involved. Studies have found large amounts of PAHs in processed yerba maté leaves[70,72,73] and high concentrations of urinary markers of PAHs in maté drinkers.[74] Maté has also been shown to have mutagenic effects in bacterial assays and to cause chromosomal aberrations in human peripheral lymphocytes treated ex vivo.[75] These lines of evidence, in addition to finding associations between maté drinking and smoking-related cancers in other organs (lung,[76] larynx,[77] oral cavity and oropharynx,[78] kidney,[79] and bladder[80,81]) suggest that PAHs may play an important role. Further evaluation of the role of PAHs in the carcinogenicity of maté is of public health significance[69] because the PAH content of maté can potentially be modified.

The large majority of EC cases in high-risk regions of South America are ESCC; there is no evidence yet with which to evaluate the association between maté drinking and EA.

Hot Foods and Drinks

Although recurrent thermal injury from intake of hot foods and drinks has long been hypothesized as a cause of EC,[4] it is still unclear whether this association exists. Some have doubted a causal association because of its biologic implausibility. For example, in 1956 Steiner suggested that the temperature of hot foods and drinks fall so rapidly in the upper digestive tract that they cannot cause injury to the esophageal mucosa.[82] However, later De Jong and colleagues[83] showed that intake of hot drinks could substantially increase the intraesophageal temperature, and this increase was a function of the initial drinking temperature and more importantly, the size of the sip. For example, drinking 65°C coffee increased the intraesophageal temperature by 6° to 12°C, depending on the sip size.[83]

The results of epidemiologic studies have shown little consistency on the role of hot drinks in esophageal carcinogenesis. Around 50 case-control studies and two cohort studies have investigated the association of drinking hot tea (green, black, and other types), coffee, maté, and other hot foods and drinks with EC. Except for maté, for which most studies have shown an increased risk, other hot drinks have been found to be associated with EC only in a minority of studies. There are several problems in establishing or refuting an association between hot drinks and EC:

1. Most of the evidence comes from case-control studies, which are prone to several biases, including recall bias and interviewer bias.
2. In some studies, consuming various types of hot drinks have been asked or analyzed together.
3. Little has been done to measure sip size or the actual temperature of the drinks—at best, the study questionnaire has asked whether the study participants drink their tea or coffee hot, warm, or cold, which may not produce reliable results.
4. These drinks have chemicals that may cause or prevent cancer, which may confound the effect of thermal irritation.

To overcome some of these problems, an ongoing cohort study in northern Iran has measured the tea drinking temperature in approximately 50,000 subjects, but the data are not available yet.[59]

Consumption of Carbonated Soft Drinks

It has been suggested that carbonated soft drinks may have contributed to the rising incidence of EA, because these drinks are acidic and may increase reflux by causing gastric distension.[84] Also, per capita consumption of these drinks increased approximately 20 years before the rise of EA rates.[84] However, case-control studies have found no association[85,86] or even an inverse association[87] between consuming soft drinks and EA risk. Likewise, case-control studies have found no association[87,88] or an inverse association[87] between soft drink consumption and ESCC risk. Therefore, the current data show no evidence that soft drinks increase EA or ESCC risk.

Consumption of Pickled Vegetables

Eating pickled vegetables was once very common in high-risk areas of China and was thought to be a major risk factor for EC in those areas.[89] As reviewed by Yang,[89] ecological studies showed higher risk of EC in areas that used higher amounts of pickled vegetables. Fungi and yeasts grow in pickled vegetables and they may release potentially carcinogenic compounds such as N-nitrosamines, Roussin red methyl ester, and mycotoxins.[89–91] Studies show that samples of pickled vegetables are mutagenic in the Ames test, can cause sister chromatid exchanges in Syrian hamster, and can also cause cancer when fed to rats.[89,92,93] However, the results of epidemiologic studies have been inconsistent. Whereas some case-control studies have shown an association between pickled vegetable intake and EC,[94–99] typically with relative risks of two to three, other case-control or cohort studies have shown no association.[12,100,101] Lack of a consistent association could partly be due to the fact that in the past the large majority of people in some high-risk areas ate pickled vegetables, which might have resulted in lack of variance. Also, a public health campaign by the government of China, which aimed to reduce pickled vegetable consumption, may have led to reporting bias in high-risk populations subject to the campaign. Therefore, further investigation of this hypothesis may be of interest. It is noteworthy that an IARC evaluation in 1993 concluded that traditional Asian pickled vegetables are possibly carcinogenic to humans (Group 2B).[102]

NUTRITIONAL DEFICIENCIES
Low Intake of Fresh Fruit and Vegetables

Low intake of fresh fruit and vegetables has long been considered as a possible risk factor for EC. A review of the evidence by World Cancer Research Fund and American Institute for Cancer Research (WCRF-AICR),[103] published in 2007, identified four cohort studies (all from China), 36 case-control studies, and seven ecological studies of the association of fruit intake and EC. The large majority of these studies found inverse associations between intake of fruits, especially citrus fruits, and EC risk. These protective associations were stronger in the case-control studies. The panel concluded that "the evidence ... though mostly from case-control studies, is consistent with a dose-response relationship... Fruits probably protect against esophageal cancer." The WCRF-AICR panel also identified five cohort studies, 37 case-control studies, and six ecological studies that had investigated the association of nonstarchy vegetables and esophageal cancer. Most case-control studies found inverse associations but cohort studies, which were mostly from China, overall found a weak inverse association. The panel's final comment was: "Nonstarchy vegetables probably protect against esophageal cancer."[103]

Since the WCRF-AICR review was conducted, at least three additional cohort studies have published their results on fruit and vegetable intake and risk of EC.[104–106] The results of all three of these cohort studies provided support for a protective association of both fruit and vegetable intake with EC.[104–106] Putting all evidence together, high intake of fruit and vegetables probably decreases EC risk by approximately 20% per 50 g of fruit or vegetable intake per day.[103]

The large majority of data on the association of fruit and vegetable intake with risk of EC comes from studies that have mainly investigated ESCC, so the results of these studies may apply only to ESCC. To our knowledge, only one cohort study has had a large enough number of ESCC and EA cases to study the effect of fruits and vegetables on these tumor types separately.[104] This study found decreased risk of ESCC, but not EA, associated with higher intake of both fruit and vegetables.

Vitamin and Mineral Deficiencies

By the early 1980s, both epidemiologists and basic scientists had obtained intriguing evidence that vitamin and micronutrient deficiencies may play important roles in the etiology of EC and several other cancers. Low intake of fruit and vegetables, which contain vitamins, were inversely associated with EC risk in most studies conducted until then. In vitro studies had shown that the antioxidant effects of some vitamins could prevent tumor formation; and people in some areas with very high-risk of EC, such as Linxian (a county in the Taihang mountains region of China), had severe deficiencies in some vitamins and minerals.[107] These findings led investigators to conduct of two large chemoprevention trials in Linxian. One of these studies, the Linxian Dysplasia Trial, randomized approximately 3,300 subjects cytologically diagnosed with esophageal squamous dysplasia (ESD) to receive a combination of 26 vitamins and minerals or a placebo.[107] The other trial, the Linxian General Population Trial, enrolled approximately 30,000 people from Linxian to test four nutrient factors: Factor A (retinol, zinc), Factor B (riboflavin, niacin), Factor C (ascorbic acid, molybdenum), and Factor D (selenium, α-tocopherol, β-carotene).[109] There was no risk reduction for EC in either trial using any of these nutritional supplements after 5 to 6 years of intervention. Longer term follow-up (through 10 years after ending the intervention) in the General Population Trial, however, showed Factor D reduced EC risk in younger subjects by 17% but increased risk in older individuals by 14%.[110] These findings, along with disappointing overall mortality and cancer incidence results from some other vitamin chemoprevention trials[111,112] and the results of some meta-analyses[113,114] have largely discouraged scientists from pursing the micronutrient hypotheses further. However, selenium and zinc deficiency may play a role in the etiology of ESCC.

Selenium deficiency has been shown to be a risk factor for upper gastrointestinal tract cancers. Both observational and experimental studies have shown that higher selenium status reduces the risk of esophageal and gastric cancers in selenium deficient populations.[108,115–117] In the Linxian General Population Trial, Factor D, which included selenium, reduced overall mortality, morality from gastric cancer, and also mortality from EC in younger individuals.[110] And, in another randomized chemoprevention trial in Linxian, selenium increased regression and reduced progression of mild ESD.[118]

Zinc deficiency enhances the effects of N-nitrosomethylbenzylamine and certain other nitrosamines in esophageal carcinogenesis in rodents.[119,120] Tissue zinc is perhaps the most relevant measure of zinc in relation to carcinogenesis.[121] The only human study investigating the association between tissue zinc and EC showed that there was a significant dose-response relationship between lower levels of zinc and increased risk of EC.[121]

MEDICATIONS
Nonsteroidal Anti-Inflammatory Drugs

A meta-analysis of nine studies, published in 2003, concluded that aspirin and other NSAIDs reduced risk of EC in a dose-response manner. More frequent use was associated with lower risk, with an overall risk reduction of approximately 40%.[122] This meta-analysis also showed that these drugs had similar inverse associations with ESCC and EA. Several other studies published since then, mostly focused on EA, have shown similar results.[123–127] This association may be due to reverse causation; people with a history of upper gastrointestinal symptoms, who are also at higher risk of cancer, may limit their use of aspirin and other NSAIDs. However, some studies stratified their results by having or not having upper gastrointestinal disorders and did not find a difference in results in these two groups of patients.[127] If the associations are causal, aspirin and NSAIDs may reduce risk by reducing inflammation and affecting the inflammation-metaplasia-cancer sequence at its early stages.[124]

Results of a short-term randomized trial in Linxian showed that celecoxib did not have any effect on regression or progression of ESD.[118] The protective effect of aspirin against the progression of BE to EA is being tested in a large, long-term trial.[128]

Medications that Relax the Lower Esophageal Sphincter

Reflux of acid from the stomach to the esophagus is usually blocked by the LES. Certain medications such as asthma drugs (β-adrenergic agonists and drugs containing theophylline), calcium channel blockers, nitroglycerin, and benzodiazepines relax the LES; hence, they may promote acid reflux and higher risk of BE and EA. The fact that use of many of the aforementioned treatments increased rapidly after the mid-1950s and the plausibility of their relation to reflux and EA led to the hypothesis that these treatments may be responsible for the EA epidemic that started in the mid-1970s.[129]

Case-control studies, however, have provided conflicting results. Whereas some studies have found no overall association with LES-relaxing drugs[126,130] others have shown increased overall BE or EA risk.[125,131,132] Among these studies, some showed increased risk with only one or two groups of medications. For example, although Vaughan and colleagues[130] found no overall association, they found increased EA risk with β-adrenergic agonists. The most consistent association was seen with asthma medications, but this association may be confounded by acid reflux, which causes both asthma and EA.[133] Other subgroup analyses have suggested that only younger individuals may be susceptible.[131] Overall the results are not entirely consistent and further studies are warranted.

Histamine₂ Receptor Antagonists

H_2 receptor antagonists (H_2 blockers), such as cimetidine and ranitidine, are a class of drugs that reduce acid production in the stomach. These drugs were first marketed in 1977 and have been highly prescribed since then. On the one hand, these medications may reduce EA risk by reducing the acid content of gastroesophageal reflux. On the other hand, they may increase EA risk by neutralizing the gastric pH, which allows bacteria to proliferate in the stomach and may result in increased production of carcinogens such as nitrosamines and acetaldehyde. In addition, cimetidine can be nitrosated in the stomach to form nitrosocimetidine, which has a chemical structure similar to the potent carcinogen N-methyl-N'-nitro-N-nitrosoguanidine.[134] At least five epidemiologic studies have investigated the association of H_2 blocker use with EC but the results are inconclusive.[135–139] Two of these studies showed increased risk of EC[136] or EA[139] with H_2 blocker use; but they did not adjust for acid reflux symptoms, which are important indications for using these treatments. Two other studies that adjusted for acid reflux symptoms found a statistically nonsignificant increased risk of EA, but they acknowledged that this nonsignificant increase might have been due to residual confounding from acid reflux.[135,137] Another study from Sweden classified the results by indication of medication use and found an increased risk of EA in the group that received H_2 blockers for "esophageal indications," rather than other indications, suggesting that the increased risk was confounded.[138] Only one of these studies[137] looked for an association between H_2 blockers and ESCC, and it did not find an association.

INFECTIONS
Helicobacter Pylori

Helicobacter pylori is a known cause of noncardia gastric adenocarcinoma and gastric mucosa-associated lymphoid tissue lymphoma.[140] The association of this gram-negative bacterium with other gastrointestinal cancers, most notably EC, has also been evaluated in several studies.

H pylori has shown a consistent pattern of association with EA. The large majority of epidemiologic studies have found a protective association, and the results of three recently published meta-analyses showed that *H pylori* colonization of the stomach is associated with a nearly 50% reduction in risk.[141–143] One of these meta-analyses also tested and showed an inverse association of *H pylori* with BE.[142] *H pylori* may decrease risk of EA by reducing gastric acid production, hence reducing acid reflux from the stomach to the esophagus.[144] It may also reduce EA risk by decreasing the production of ghrelin, a hormone that is mostly produced in the stomach and stimulates appetite.[145] A reduction in the level of ghrelin may lead to lower rates of obesity, an important risk factor for EA.[40]

In the past few decades, advances in sanitation and the widespread use of antibiotics have caused a rapid decline in *H pylori* colonization prevalence in human populations,[146] especially in Western countries. In the United States, for example, data from the National Health and Nutritional Examination Survey 1999–2000 indicated the presence of *H pylori* in only 5% of children who were born in the 1990s.[147] This was far lower than that seen in older people of the United States[147] or in children of other countries with lower socioeconomic status.[148] Therefore, it is conceivable that the steep decline in *H pylori* colonization rates in the past few decades may be partly responsible for the recent increase in EA incidence in Western countries.

In contrast to its association with EA, *H pylori* has not shown a consistent association with ESCC. Whereas some studies have found a two-fold increased risk of ESCC with *H pylori* colonization in the stomach,[98,149] others have found no association[150] or even reduced risk.[151] Three recent meta-analyses that summarized the association of *H pylori* with ESCC found no overall association, with summary odds ratios very close to unity, but they showed substantial heterogeneity in results of the published studies.[141–143]

Human Papillomavirus

Oncogenic types of HPV, most notably HPV 16 and HPV 18, are necessary causes of cervical cancer,[152,153] and play an important role in the etiology of the epithelial cancers of the vulva, anus, penis, and oropharyngeal cavity.[153,154] However, despite 25 years of research and well over 100 studies of EC, the role of HPV in the etiology of this cancer remains controversial.[153]

HPV was first suspected to have a role in the etiology of EC in 1982, when histologic findings suggesting the presence of HPV were observed in benign esophageal epithelia and malignant esophageal tumors.[155] Since then, two major approaches have been used to investigate a possible role of HPV in causing EC: (1) searching for the presence of HPV DNA in tumors using polymerase chain reaction (PCR) and (2) comparing cases and controls in case-control or cohort studies for serum antibodies against HPV. PCR-based methods can detect DNA from the carcinogenic HPV types in nearly all cervical cancers.[153] In contrast, PCR results have been very inconsistent in esophageal cancers.[153,156] While many studies have found no evidence of HPV in esophageal tumors,[157–163] others have found HPV in up to 75%.[164] This inconsistency may be due to true geographic variation,[156] or it may simply reflect contamination during sample preparation or conducting the PCR. The results of case-control or cohort studies that have used serologic assays against HPV virus-like particles have also been inconsistent. Whereas some studies have found very strong (relative risks of five or more),[165,166] moderate-to-strong (relative risks of two–five),[167] or weak (relative risks of one–two) associations between HPV 16 or HPV 18 and EC, others have found no association[168–170] or even inverse associations. The inconsistency of these results may be due to differences in study design (case-control versus cohort studies), geographic variation (high-risk versus low-risk areas), differences in positivity cutpoints used in different studies, lack of appropriate adjustment for tobacco use or alcohol consumption, or simply chance fluctuation due to the small number of cases in some studies. Efforts to find the source of heterogeneity have so far been inconclusive.[170] Because of these conflicting results, a recent report by IARC concluded that "there is inadequate evidence in humans for carcinogenicity of HPV in the esophagus."[153]

CHEMICAL CARCINOGENS
Polycyclic Aromatic Hydrocarbons

PAHs are produced during incomplete combustion of organic materials. The major sources of exposure to PAHs are smoking tobacco,[42] eating charbroiled meat and other food products,[171] air pollution,[172] and occupational exposure.[173]

PAHs have long been suspected to be human carcinogens. In 1755, Percivall Pott[174] found that exposure to soot, which contains high amounts of PAHs, causes scrotal cancers in chimney sweeps. In 1915, Yamagiwa, a Japanese pathologist, induced cancer for the first time by applying coal to the ears of rabbits.[175] Kennaway and colleagues[175] at Royal Cancer Hospital in London found dibenz(a,h)anthracene and benzo[a]pyrene, two PAHs, to be the active carcinogenic compounds in coal tar capable of inducing skin cancer in mice.

A causal link between PAHs or PAH-containing substances and cancer has been established for cancers of the skin, lung, and bladder.[176] Tobacco smoke, which contains significant amounts of PAHs, is causally linked to EC. However, evidence linking other PAH-containing substances or individual PAHs to EC is based only on ecologic studies and is therefore circumstantial. Studies in Linxian have shown histopathologic evidence in EC cases consistent with high exposure to PAHs,[177] presence of high levels of carcinogenic PAHs in staple foods,[178] and high concentrations of urinary markers of PAHs.[179] Studies in Golestan Province of Iran have also shown very high concentrations of urinary markers of PAHs in a majority of the residents.[180] Therefore, further evaluation of this association is of significant interest. Evaluating the association of PAHs with EC or other cancers, however, has proven difficult, partly because there are no valid and reliable markers of long-term PAH exposure that can be used in epidemiologic studies. Urinary markers of PAHs reflect exposure only in the 24 to 72 hours before urine collection.[181] Using PAH-DNA adducts or PAH-protein adducts as markers of exposure in epidemiologic studies have also been hampered by other limitations, such as lack of sensitivity to low exposures, nonlinearity at high exposures, use of surrogate tissues (such as blood lymphocytes) instead of the target tissue of interest, and high cell turnover rates in many tissues, which make it impossible to measure long-term exposure.[182,183] Nevertheless, adducts have been useful in establishing causal links between some carcinogens and cancer, such as the causal relationship between tobacco smoking and cervical cancer, and better assays may help future research evaluation of a PAH link to EC.

N-Nitroso Compounds

N-nitroso compounds (NNCs) are strong animal carcinogens and have been shown to cause cancers of the nasal cavity, esophagus, and stomach in several animal models.[184–187] The role of these compounds as human carcinogens is less well established.

The relevance of NNCs to human cancer has been difficult to assess because humans are exposed to these compounds in many different ways and because no valid and long-term integrated biomarker of exposure has been developed. Humans can be exposed to NNCs from tobacco smoking, occupational exposure, and many food sources[188] and also from endogenous synthesis, which contributes to 45% to 75% of the total exposure.[189] Nitrosamines and nitrosamides, two major subgroups of NNCs, are formed by the endogenous reaction of nitrites with amines or amides, respectively. Nitrites are directly found in sodium nitrite and various foods, and are also formed by reduction of ingested or salivary nitrates.[190–192] Vegetables are the main sources of exogenous nitrates but high levels of nitrates may also be found in water.[192] Reduction of nitrates to nitrites by oral bacteria is a major contributor to the formation of NCCs and may be one of the reasons why poor oral health has been associated with higher risk of EC and gastric cancer.[193,194] To date, no NNC-DNA adducts are available that are easily measurable and accurately represent long-term exposure to NNCs.

Despite these challenges, there is some indirect evidence linking NNCs to EC. Jakszyn and Gonzalez[195] recently conducted a systematic review of case-control and cohort studies associating nitrosamine exposure and foods that are direct or indirect sources of these compounds with EC risk, and found that eating processed meat, a major source of nitrites and nitrosamines, was consistently associated with higher risk of EC.[195]

Acetaldehyde

Humans can be exposed to acetaldehyde in several ways, most notably by drinking alcohol. Ethanol is converted to acetaldehyde by alcohol dehydrogenase (ADH) enzymes and then to acetate by acetaldehyde dehydrogenase (ALDH) enzymes.[196] Therefore, higher alcohol consumption and genetic polymorphisms that enhance the activity of ADHs or decrease the activity of ALDHs result in higher acetaldehyde exposure.[196] In addition to drinking alcohol, humans are exposed to acetaldehyde by smoking cigarettes, eating moldy food, burning wood and coal, and also by in vivo metabolism of sugars by oral and colonic bacteria.[197,198] In vitro, acetaldehyde causes point mutations in human lymphocytes, sister chromatic exchanges, cellular proliferation, and inhibits DNA repair. In 1999, the IARC[197] classified acetaldehyde as a known carcinogen for animals but only a possible carcinogen for humans, mostly because there was little human data at the time. Since then, genetic polymorphisms in ADH genes and ALDH2 that favor the accumulation of acetaldehyde have been observed to increase ESCC risk,[196] thus adding to the evidence of acetaldehyde carcinogenicity in humans. In addition, acetaldehyde may link drinking alcohol, smoking tobacco, eating moldy foods, and poor oral health to ESCC.[198] Therefore, further studies in humans are warranted.

Fumonisins

Fumonisins are toxins secreted from *Fusarium verticillioides* (formerly *Fusarium moniliforme*), a fungus that grows mostly on maize. Fumonisin B$_1$ is a known animal carcinogen and has been shown to cause tumors of the liver and kidney in mice and rats.[199,200] Evidence for the carcinogenicity of fumonisins in humans, however, is circumstantial, and is mostly limited to ecologic studies. Ecologic studies in China, Iran, and South Africa have shown higher exposure to fumonisins in areas with higher risk of EC.[201–203] The only case-control study that examined fumonisin exposure in relation to EC risk was conducted in Linxian, China, and found no association between exposure and risk.[204] However, the biomarkers of exposure used in this study were of uncertain value and the results were not conclusive. Further epidemiologic studies are needed to establish or refute an association between fumonisins and EC.

PREDISPOSING CONDITIONS
Gastroesophageal Acid Reflux

Symptomatic gastroesophageal acid reflux is perhaps the strongest known risk factor for EA. In a population-based case-control study from Sweden, Lagergren and colleagues[205] showed a strong dose-response association of both frequency and duration of reflux with EA. In this study, any reflux was associated with approximately eight-fold increased risk, but risk was increased up to 20-fold in those with very frequent and severe reflux.[205] Several other studies published since then have confirmed a dose-response association between reflux and EA,[39,40,137,206] but the relative risks have been almost half as strong as those reported in Lagergren's original study (approximately four-fold overall and eight-fold for those having the highest frequencies).

Consistency of the results across studies, dose-response relationship, and strength of association all implicate a causal relationship between reflux and EA. There is also a strong association between acid reflux and BE.[207] Recurrent acid reflux may cause EA by inducing metaplasia in the mucosa of the lower part of the esophagus and changing the local squamous tissue into BE. Unlike EA, ESCC is not caused by acid reflux.

Obesity

Two meta-analyses[208,209] have summarized the association of overweight (body mass index from 25 to < 30 kg/m^2) and obesity (body mass index of 30 kg/m^2 or higher) with EA. The more recent of these two[209] identified 14 studies and found that EA risk increased approximately two-fold to three-fold in overweight and obese individuals. It also observed a dose-response relationship; risk was slightly higher in obese than in overweight people. Since the publication of this meta-analysis, several additional population-based or cohort studies of obesity and EA risk have been published, which have also shown two- to three-fold increased risks and dose-response relationships.[39,40,210,211]

Since this association is consistent across a large number of studies, is moderately strong, and has a dose-response pattern, it is highly likely that it is causal. In fact, increasing weight trends in the United States and other Western countries may be partially responsible for increasing incidence rates of EA in these countries. Several mechanisms have been suggested to explain the causal link.[212] Obesity increases intra-abdominal pressure which in turn could increase risk of gastroesophageal reflux and BE. In fact, obesity has been convincingly linked to GERD,[208,213] and measures of central obesity, such as waist-to-hip ratio and abdominal circumference, have been linked to BE.[214,215] In addition, adipose tissue is physiologically active and may increase risk by way of modulation of levels of polypeptides such as ghrelin, leptin, adiponectin, and insulin-like growth factors.[212]

Hiatal Hernia

Hiatal hernia can increase EA risk by increasing gastroesophageal acid reflux. Many studies have investigated the association of hiatal hernia with EA, and all have found increased risks, with relative risks ranging from two-fold to six-fold.[135,137,138,206] Also, among people with BE, having a large hiatal hernia increases the risk of high grade dysplasia and EA.[216,217] In contrast to EA, the risk of ESCC is not increased by the presence of a hiatal hernia.

Achalasia

Achalasia is a motility disorder of the esophagus characterized by aperistalsis in the distal esophagus and loss of LES relaxation. This leads to stasis and fermentation of food in the esophagus, which may cause increased inflammation and higher EC risk.[218]

Most case series have reported EC in 3% to 7% of achalasia patients,[219] which is far higher than the rates seen in normal population. Follow-up studies of achalasia patients have consistently shown substantially increased risk of EC,[220–223] but because the size of achalasia cohorts have been small, different magnitudes of relative risks have been reported. One of the largest of these cohorts that has had a long-term follow-up is conducted in Sweden. The latest results from this cohort[223] showed a 10-fold increased risk of both ESCC and EA in achalasia patients compared with the rest of the population.

Substantial increases in risk of EC have also been reported in patients with other benign diseases that cause esophageal obstruction, including patients with esophageal webs and lye stricture.[224]

Gastric Atrophy

Atrophy of the gastric mucosa has long been known to be a precursor lesion for gastric cancer.[225] However, an association between gastric atrophy and ESCC is a relatively recent finding.

A Swedish study showed for the first time that pernicious anemia patients had a three-fold higher risk of ESCC than the general population.[226,227] Because a main feature of pernicious anemia is gastric atrophy, it was hypothesized that gastric atrophy may also cause ESCC.

Gastric atrophy can be detected either by direct histologic examination of gastric biopsies or by measuring serum pepsinogens, proenzymes that are secreted by the gastric epithelial cells; low serum pepsinogen I (PGI) or low serum pepsinogen I/pepsinogen II (PGI/II) ratio indicate atrophy.[228,229] Ye and colleagues[230] published the first case-control evaluation of the association between serum pepsinogens and ESCC risk and found a four-fold increased risk of ESCC in patients with low serum PGI. These findings were confirmed by a case-control study from Japan that found gastric atrophy, diagnosed serologically or histologically, was associated with a four-fold or greater increased risk of superficial ESCC.[231] Also, a case-control study from Linxian showed an almost linear association between the lower serum PGI/II and risk of ESD.[232] A recent study from Netherlands found that patients with gastric atrophy had a two-fold higher risk of ESCC than the general population[233] but ESCC risk did not increase with increasing severity of atrophy, which suggested that the association of gastric atrophy and ESCC may be confounded by other factors such as smoking. There is no evidence for an increased risk of EA associated with atrophy.[227,230]

How can gastric atrophy increase the risk of ESCC? Because gastric glands disappear in atrophy, acid secretion is reduced, which results in a proliferation of bacteria in the stomach.[234] These bacteria, in turn, may increase the production of carcinogens such as nitrosamines and acetaldehyde, which may explain the association between gastric atrophy and gastric and esophageal neoplasia.

Poor Oral Hygiene and Tooth Loss

Like several other etiologic hypotheses, the hypothesis that poor oral health could potentially be a risk factor for EC dates back at least seven decades.[3,88] American physicians earlier in this century suggested that patients with EC had poorer dental hygiene than the general population.[3] Chinese scientists also found that the prevalence of dental caries was higher in people from high-risk areas than other Chinese people, and oral hygiene was poorer in patients with EC or ESD than other people (reviewed by CS Yang).[89] More recently, a long-term prospective cohort study conducted in Linxian showed that tooth loss was associated with a small but statistically significant increase in ESCC risk (relative risk of 1.3, comparing greater versus less than median).[193,235] Subsequent case-control studies in South America,[236] Central Europe,[235] Japan,[237] and Iran[238] also showed that tooth loss was associated with a two-fold to three-fold increased risk of EC. Furthermore, other studies from China and Iran showed a significantly increased risk of ESD associated with poor oral health.[239,240]

The associations found between tooth loss or poor oral hygiene with EC could be confounded by smoking, alcohol consumption, low socioeconomic status, or other factors. Some of the aforementioned studies have extensively addressed these issues. For example, Abnet and colleagues[238] examined the associations in people who never smoked or drank and the results did not change materially. Other issues still exist. In some studies, clear dose-response associations were not observed and, in some, associations were seen with some markers of oral health but not with others. In a small study in Finland, no association was seen between tooth loss and EC risk.[194] Nevertheless, the accumulated data are definitely intriguing.

If these associations are indeed causal, there are several mechanistic hypotheses:[194]

  Changes in oral microbial flora which result in both poor oral health and in increased production of carcinogens such as nitrosamines and acetaldehyde
  Physical irritation and damage to the esophageal epithelium due to swallowing unchewed food
  Change in dietary patterns and nutrient intake due to poor dentition
  Infection of the esophageal mucosa with an oral microorganism
  Genetic factors that affect both oral health and EC.

Among these, the first proposed mechanism seems most intriguing and could be tested in several ways; for example by comparing nitrosamine and acetaldehyde production among people with and without ESD.

Nearly all studies of the association between poor oral health and EC risk have been done in areas that ESCC constitutes the large majority of the cases, so the results are most relevant to ESCC. To date, there have been no studies specifically evaluating an association between poor oral health and EA.

OCCUPATIONAL EXPOSURE

EC is generally not considered an occupational cancer. However, several studies have suggested that occupational exposure to asbestos could increase EC risk between 2-fold and 16-fold.[241–245] Other studies have found increased EC risk in relation to occupational exposure to silica.[246–249] However, other studies have shown no or only very slight increased risk with these occupational exposures. For example, Kang and colleagues[250] found only an 8% increased risk of EC in relation to asbestos exposure. Further research is required in this area.

IARC has classified crystalline silica and asbestos as carcinogenic to humans (Group 1 carcinogen), mostly because of their effect in causing lung cancer and mesothelioma.[251,252]

LOW SOCIOECONOMIC STATUS

It has long been known that EC is a disease of the poor and the socially disadvantaged. In his 1939 paper, Watson[4] writes "... it should be noted that a large percentage of the patients in this series [of 771 EC cases] are ... of a station in life definitely below average, and further, that 9 out of 10 patients with this disease are in the lower middle class socially, and on the whole financially insecure."

Since then, a large number of epidemiologic studies have confirmed that EC risk is higher in populations with lower socioeconomic status (SES).[12,29,31,51,240,253–260] These studies have had different designs (case-control, cohort, and comparisons of incident cases with the general population), used different SES indicators (eg, income and education), and were from all parts of the world (North America, Europe, East and South Asia, the Middle East, and Africa). Therefore, the finding that EC is more common in lower SES groups is nearly universal.

It is difficult to assign an approximate relative risk to SES, partly because SES itself is not a well-defined entity, and various SES indicators, such as education and income, may have different meanings in different populations. However, using various indicators, most studies have reported an increased risk of two-fold to four-fold among those with lower compared with those with higher SES.

Low education and low income are not direct biologic causes of EC. Attempts have been made to identify more direct causal mechanisms, such as higher use of tobacco or alcohol or poorer nutrition among people with lower SES. However, these attempts have not yielded consistent results.

The majority of studies of SES and EC have been conducted in populations with high-risk of ESCC, so there is little doubt that ESCC is inversely associated with SES. There is less data available for EA; three recent studies suggested that SES is inversely associated with EA too,[31,256,257] but one study did not find an association.[261]

SUMMARY

Over the past century, a large number of factors have been tested for their potential association with EC risk. Whereas older studies mainly investigated the etiology of ESCC, the newer studies in Western countries have also investigated the causes of EA.

The results of these studies have established excessive use of alcohol, tobacco use, low intake of fresh fruit and vegetables, low SES, and drinking maté as risk factors for ESCC. Also, certain physiologic or pathologic conditions, such as gastric atrophy and achalasia, may predispose people to higher risk of ESCC. There are other potential but as yet unsubstantiated risk factors. For example, PAHs and acetaldehyde may play an important role in the etiology of ESCC in high-risk areas of Iran or China, but this remains to be verified in future studies.

Three important risk factors have been identified for EA: gastroesophageal acid reflux, obesity, and smoking. Absence of *H pylori* in the stomach is also becoming increasingly recognized as a risk factor. Other factors, such as the use of LES-relaxing medications need to be further studied.

REFERENCES

1. Kamangar F, Dores GM, Anderson WF. Patterns of cancer incidence, mortality, and prevalence across five continents: defining priorities to reduce cancer disparities in different geographic regions of the world. J Clin Oncol 2006; 24(14):2137–50.
2. Parkin DM, Bray F, Ferlay J, et al. Global cancer statistics, 2002. CA Cancer J Clin 2005;55(2):74–108.
3. Craver LF. Clinical study of etiology of gastric and esophageal carcinoma. Am J Cancer 1932;16(1):68–102.
4. Watson WL. Cancer of the esophagus: some etiological considerations. Am J Roentgenol 1939;41(3):420–4.
5. Blot WJ, Devesa SS, Kneller RW, et al. Rising incidence of adenocarcinoma of the esophagus and gastric cardia. JAMA 1991;265(10):1287–9.
6. Brown LM, Devesa SS, Chow WH. Incidence of adenocarcinoma of the esophagus among white Americans by sex, stage, and age. J Natl Cancer Inst 2008;100:1184–7.
7. Botterweck AA, Schouten LJ, Volovics A, et al. Trends in incidence of adenocarcinoma of the oesophagus and gastric cardia in ten European countries. Int J Epidemiol 2000;29(4):645–54.
8. Vizcaino AP, Moreno V, Lambert R, et al. Time trends incidence of both major histologic types of esophageal carcinomas in selected countries, 1973–1995. Int J Cancer 2002;99(6):860–8.
9. van Blankenstein M, Looman CW, Siersema PD, et al. Trends in the incidence of adenocarcinoma of the oesophagus and cardia in the Netherlands 1989–2003. Br J Cancer 2007;96(11):1767–71.
10. Corley DA, Buffler PA. Oesophageal and gastric cardia adenocarcinomas: analysis of regional variation using the cancer incidence in five continents database. Int J Epidemiol 2001;30(6):1415–25.
11. Islami F, Kamangar F, Aghcheli K, et al. Epidemiologic features of upper gastrointestinal tract cancer in northeastern Iran. Br J Cancer 2004;90(7):1402–6.
12. Tran GD, Sun XD, Abnet CC, et al. Prospective study of risk factors for esophageal and gastric cancers in the Linxian general population trial cohort in China. Int J Cancer 2005;113(3):456–63.
13. Munoz N, Day NE. Esophageal cancer. In: Schottenfeld D, Fraumeni JF, editors. Cancer epidemiology and prevention. 2nd edition. New York: Oxford University Press; 1996. p. 681–706.
14. Ke L. Mortality and incidence trends from esophagus cancer in selected geographic areas of China circa 1970–90. Int J Cancer 2002;102(3):271–4.
15. Mahboubi E, Kmet J, Cook PJ, et al. Oesophageal cancer studies in the Caspian Littoral of Iran: the Caspian Cancer Registry. Br J Cancer 1973;28(3):197–214.
16. Wang GQ, Abnet CC, Shen Q, et al. Histological precursors of oesophageal squamous cell carcinoma: results from a 13 year prospective follow up study in a high risk population. Gut 2005;54(2):187–92.
17. Shaheen NJ, Crosby MA, Bozymski EM, et al. Is there publication bias in the reporting of cancer risk in Barrett's esophagus? Gastroenterology 2000;119(2):333–8.
18. Jankowski JA, Provenzale D, Moayyedi P. Esophageal adenocarcinoma arising from Barrett's metaplasia has regional variations in the west. Gastroenterology 2002;122(2):588–90.
19. US Department of Health, Education, and Welfare (DHEW). Smoking and health: a report of the Surgeon General. Washington, DC: US Government Press Office; 1979.

20. US Department of Health and Human Services (USDHHS). Reducing the health consequences of smoking: 25 years of progress: a report of the Surgeon General. Washington, DC: US Government Press Office; 1989.
21. Carstensen JM, Pershagen G, Eklund G. Mortality in relation to cigarette and pipe smoking: 16 years' observation of 25,000 Swedish men. J Epidemiol Community Health 1987;41(2):166–72.
22. Doll R, Peto R, Wheatley K, et al. Mortality in relation to smoking: 40 years' observations on male British doctors. BMJ 1994;309(6959):901–11.
23. McLaughlin JK, Hrubec Z, Blot WJ, et al. Smoking and cancer mortality among U.S. veterans: a 26-year follow-up. Int J Cancer 1995;60(2):190–3.
24. Ishikawa A, Kuriyama S, Tsubono Y, et al. Smoking, alcohol drinking, green tea consumption and the risk of esophageal cancer in Japanese men. J Epidemiol 2006;16(5):185–92.
25. Freedman ND, Abnet CC, Leitzmann MF, et al. A prospective study of tobacco, alcohol, and the risk of esophageal and gastric cancer subtypes. Am J Epidemiol 2007;165(12):1424–33.
26. US Department of Health and Human Services (USDHHS). The health consequences of smoking—Cancer: a report of the Surgeon General. Washington, DC: US Government Press Office; 1982.
27. International Agency for Research on Cancer. Betel-quid and areca-nut chewing and some areca-nut derived nitrosamines. IARC Monogr Eval Carcinog Risks Hum 2004;85:1–334.
28. Nasrollahzadeh D, Kamangar F, Aghcheli K, et al. Opium, tobacco, and alcohol use in relation to oesophageal squamous cell carcinoma in a high-risk area of Iran. Br J Cancer 2008;98(11):1857–63.
29. Cook-Mozaffari PJ, Azordegan F, Day NE, et al. Oesophageal cancer studies in the Caspian Littoral of Iran: results of a case-control study. Br J Cancer 1979; 39(3):293–309.
30. Kamangar F, Malekzadeh R, Dawsey SM, et al. Esophageal cancer in Northeastern Iran: a review. Arch Iran Med 2007;10(1):70–82.
31. Brown LM, Silverman DT, Pottern LM, et al. Adenocarcinoma of the esophagus and esophagogastric junction in white men in the United States: alcohol, tobacco, and socioeconomic factors. Cancer Causes Control 1994;5(4):333–40.
32. Vaughan TL, Davis S, Kristal A, et al. Obesity, alcohol, and tobacco as risk factors for cancers of the esophagus and gastric cardia: adenocarcinoma versus squamous cell carcinoma. Cancer Epidemiol Biomarkers Prev 1995; 4(2):85–92.
33. Gammon MD, Schoenberg JB, Ahsan H, et al. Tobacco, alcohol, and socioeconomic status and adenocarcinomas of the esophagus and gastric cardia. J Natl Cancer Inst 1997;89(17):1277–84.
34. Lagergren J, Bergstrom R, Lindgren A, et al. The role of tobacco, snuff and alcohol use in the aetiology of cancer of the oesophagus and gastric cardia. Int J Cancer 2000;85(3):340–6.
35. Cheng KK, Sharp L, McKinney PA, et al. A case-control study of oesophageal adenocarcinoma in women: a preventable disease. Br J Cancer 2000;83(1): 127–32.
36. Wu AH, Wan P, Bernstein L. A multiethnic population-based study of smoking, alcohol and body size and risk of adenocarcinomas of the stomach and esophagus (United States). Cancer Causes Control 2001;12(8):721–32.
37. Chen H, Ward MH, Graubard BI, et al. Dietary patterns and adenocarcinoma of the esophagus and distal stomach. Am J Clin Nutr 2002;75(1):137–44.

38. Veugelers PJ, Porter GA, Guernsey DL, et al. Obesity and lifestyle risk factors for gastroesophageal reflux disease, Barrett esophagus and esophageal adenocarcinoma. Dis Esophagus 2006;19(5):321–8.
39. Anderson LA, Watson RG, Murphy SJ, et al. Risk factors for Barrett's oesophagus and oesophageal adenocarcinoma: results from the FINBAR study. World J Gastroenterol 2007;13(10):1585–94.
40. Whiteman DC, Sadeghi S, Pandeya N, et al. Combined effects of obesity, acid reflux and smoking on the risk of adenocarcinomas of the oesophagus. Gut 2007;57(2):173–80.
41. U.S. Department of Health and Human Services (USDHHS). The Health Consequences of Smoking: A report of the Surgeon General. Washington, DC: U.S. Government Press Office, 2004.
42. Danaei G, Vander HS, Lopez AD, et al. Causes of cancer in the world: comparative risk assessment of nine behavioural and environmental risk factors. Lancet 2005;366(9499):1784–93.
43. Hecht SS. Tobacco carcinogens, their biomarkers and tobacco-induced cancer. Nat Rev Cancer 2003;3(10):733–44.
44. Tuyns AJ. Cancer of the oesophagus: further evidence of the relation to drinking habits in France. Int J Cancer 1970;5(1):152–6.
45. Audigier JC, Tuyns AJ, Lambert R. Epidemiology of Oesophageal cancer in France. Increasing mortality and persistent correlation with alcoholism. Digestion 1975;13(4):209–19.
46. Tuyns AJ, Pequignot G, Abbatucci JS. Oesophageal cancer and alcohol consumption; importance of type of beverage. Int J Cancer 1979;23(4):443–7.
47. Tuyns AJ. Oesophageal cancer in non-smoking drinkers and in non-drinking smokers. Int J Cancer 1983;32(4):443–4.
48. International Agency for Research on Cancer. Alcoholic beverage consumption and ethyl carbamate (urethane). IARC Monogr Eval Carcinog Risks Hum, in press.
49. Boffetta P, Garfinkel L. Alcohol drinking and mortality among men enrolled in an American Cancer Society prospective study. Epidemiology 1990;1(5):342–8.
50. Brown LM, Hoover RN, Greenberg RS, et al. Are racial differences in squamous cell esophageal cancer explained by alcohol and tobacco use? J Natl Cancer Inst 1994;86(17):1340–5.
51. Brown LM, Hoover R, Silverman D, et al. Excess incidence of squamous cell esophageal cancer among US Black men: role of social class and other risk factors. Am J Epidemiol 2001;153(2):114–22.
52. Kabat GC, Ng SK, Wynder EL. Tobacco, alcohol intake, and diet in relation to adenocarcinoma of the esophagus and gastric cardia. Cancer Causes Control 1993;4(2):123–32.
53. Boffetta P, Hashibe M. Alcohol and cancer. Lancet Oncol 2006;7(2):149–56.
54. Ghadirian P, Stein GF, Gorodetzky C, et al. Oesophageal cancer studies in the Caspian littoral of Iran: some residual results, including opium use as a risk factor. Int J Cancer 1985;35(5):593–7.
55. Hewer T, Rose E, Ghadirian P, et al. Ingested mutagens from opium and tobacco pyrolysis products and cancer of the oesophagus. Lancet 1978;2(8088):494–6.
56. Malaveille C, Friesen M, Camus AM, et al. Mutagens produced by the pyrolysis of opium and its alkaloids as possible risk factors in cancer of the bladder and oesophagus. Carcinogenesis 1982;3(5):577–85.
57. Perry PE, Thomson EJ, Vijayalaxmi, et al. Induction of SCE by opium pyrolysates in CHO cells and human peripheral blood lymphocytes. Carcinogenesis 1983;4(2):227–30.

58. Friesen M, O'Neill IK, Malaveille C, et al. Characterization and identification of 6 mutagens in opium pyrolysates implicated in oesophageal cancer in Iran. Mutat Res 1985;150(1-2):177–91.
59. Pourshams A, Saadatian-Elahi M, Nouraie M, et al. Golestan cohort study of esophageal cancer: feasibility and first results. Br J Cancer 2004;92:176–81.
60. Victora CG, Munoz N, Horta BL, et al. Patterns of maté drinking in a Brazilian city. Cancer Res 1990;50(22):7112–5.
61. Castellsague X, Munoz N, De Stefani E, et al. Influence of maté drinking, hot beverages and diet on esophageal cancer risk in South America. Int J Cancer 2000;88(4):658–64.
62. Parkin DM, Bray FI, Devesa SS. Cancer burden in the year 2000. The global picture. Eur J Cancer 2001;37(Suppl 8):S4–66.
63. Vassallo A, Correa P, De Stefani E, et al. Esophageal cancer in Uruguay: a case-control study. J Natl Cancer Inst 1985;75(6):1005–9.
64. Victora CG, Munoz N, Day NE, et al. Hot beverages and oesophageal cancer in southern Brazil: a case-control study. Int J Cancer 1987;39(6):710–6.
65. De Stefani E, Munoz N, Esteve J, et al. Maté drinking, alcohol, tobacco, diet, and esophageal cancer in Uruguay. Cancer Res 1990;50(2):426–31.
66. Castelletto R, Castellsague X, Munoz N, et al. Alcohol, tobacco, diet, maté drinking, and esophageal cancer in Argentina. Cancer Epidemiol Biomarkers Prev 1994;3(7):557–64.
67. Rolon PA, Castellsague X, Benz M, et al. Hot and cold maté drinking and esophageal cancer in Paraguay. Cancer Epidemiol Biomarkers Prev 1995;4(6):595–605.
68. Sewram V, De Stefani E, Brennan P, et al. Maté consumption and the risk of squamous cell esophageal cancer in Uruguay. Cancer Epidemiol Biomarkers Prev 2003;12(6):508–13.
69. De Stefani E, Deneo-Pellegrini H, Ronco AL, et al. Food groups and risk of squamous cell carcinoma of the oesophagus: a case-control study in Uruguay. Br J Cancer 2003;89(7):1209–14.
70. Kamangar F, Schantz MM, Abnet CC, et al. High levels of carcinogenic polycyclic aromatic hydrocarbons in maté drinks. Cancer Epidemiol Biomarkers Prev 2008;17(5):1262–8.
71. International Agency for Research on Cancer. Coffee, tea, maté, methylxanthines and methylglyoxal. IARC Monogr Eval Carcinog Risks Hum 1991;51:1–513.
72. Ruschenburg U. Benzo[a]pyrene content of coffee and some other foodstuff. Lome. In: IIe colloque scientifique sur le cafe, Lome; 1985. p. 205–12.
73. Schlemitz S, Pfannhauser W. Supercritical fluid extraction of mononitrated polycyclic aromatic hydrocarbons from tea—correlation with PAH concentration. Z Lebensm Unters Forsch 1997;205(4):305–10.
74. Fagundes RB, Abnet CC, Strickland PT, et al. Higher urine 1- hydroxy pyrene glucuronide (1-OHPG) is associated with tobacco smoke exposure and drinking mate in healthy subjects from Rio Grande do Sul, Brazil. BMC Cancer 2006;6(1):139.
75. Fonseca CA, Otto SS, Paumgartten FJ, et al. Nontoxic, mutagenic, and clastogenic activities of Maté-Chimarrao (Ilex paraguariensis). J Environ Pathol Toxicol Oncol 2000;19(4):333–46.
76. De Stefani E, Fierro L, Correa P, et al. Maté drinking and risk of lung cancer in males: a case-control study from Uruguay. Cancer Epidemiol Biomarkers Prev 1996;5(7):515–9.

77. Pintos J, Franco EL, Oliveira BV, et al. Maté, coffee, and tea consumption and risk of cancers of the upper aerodigestive tract in southern Brazil. Epidemiology 1994;5(6):583–90.

78. Goldenberg D, Golz A, Joachims HZ. The beverage maté: a risk factor for cancer of the head and neck. Head Neck 2003;25(7):595–601.

79. De Stefani E, Fierro L, Mendilaharsu M, et al. Meat intake, 'maté' drinking and renal cell cancer in Uruguay: a case-control study. Br J Cancer 1998;78(9):1239–43.

80. De Stefani E, Boffetta P, eo-Pellegrini H, et al. Non-alcoholic beverages and risk of bladder cancer in Uruguay. BMC Cancer 2007;7:57.

81. Bates MN, Hopenhayn C, Rey OA, et al. Bladder cancer and maté consumption in Argentina: a case-control study. Cancer Lett 2007;246(1–2):268–73.

82. Steiner PE. The etiology and histogenesis of carcinoma of the esophagus. Cancer 1956;9:436–52.

83. De Jong UW, Day NE, Mounier-Kuhn PL, et al. The relationship between the ingestion of hot coffee and intraoesophageal temperature. Gut 1972;13(1): 24–30.

84. Mallath MK. Rise of esophageal adenocarcinoma in USA is temporally associated with the rise in carbonated soft drink consumption. Gastroenterology 2004;126(Suppl 2):A619.

85. Lagergren J, Viklund P, Jansson C. Carbonated soft drinks and risk of esophageal adenocarcinoma: a population-based case-control study. J Natl Cancer Inst 2006;98(16):1158–61.

86. Ibiebele TI, Hughes MC, O'Rourke P, et al. Cancers of the esophagus and carbonated beverage consumption: a population-based case-control study. Cancer Causes Control 2008;19(6):577–84.

87. Mayne ST, Risch HA, Dubrow R, et al. Carbonated soft drink consumption and risk of esophageal adenocarcinoma. J Natl Cancer Inst 2006;98(1):72–5.

88. Gallus S, Talamini R, Fernandez E, et al. Re: Carbonated soft drink consumption and risk of esophageal adenocarcinoma. J Natl Cancer Inst 2006;98(9):645–6.

89. Yang CS. Research on esophageal cancer in China: a review. Cancer Res 1980; 40(8 Pt 1):2633–44.

90. Cheng SJ, Sala M, Li MH, et al. Promoting effect of Roussin's red identified in pickled vegetables from Linxian China. Carcinogenesis 1981;2(4):313–9.

91. Zhang WX, Xu MS, Wang GH, et al. Quantitative analysis of Roussin red methyl ester in pickled vegetables. Cancer Res 1983;43(1):339–41.

92. Cheng SJ, Sala M, Li MH, et al. Mutagenic, transforming and promoting effect of pickled vegetables from Linxian county, China. Carcinogenesis 1980;1(8):685–92.

93. Lu SH, Camus AM, Tomatis L, et al. Mutagenicity of extracts of pickled vegetables collected in Linhsien County, a high-incidence area for esophageal cancer in Northern China. J Natl Cancer Inst 1981;66(1):33–6.

94. Cheng KK, Day NE, Duffy SW, et al. Pickled vegetables in the aetiology of oesophageal cancer in Hong Kong Chinese. Lancet 1992;339(8805):1314–8.

95. Hung HC, Huang MC, Lee JM, et al. Association between diet and esophageal cancer in Taiwan. J Gastroenterol Hepatol 2004;19(6):632–7.

96. Takezaki T, Gao CM, Wu JZ, et al. Dietary protective and risk factors for esophageal and stomach cancers in a low-epidemic area for stomach cancer in Jiangsu Province, China: comparison with those in a high-epidemic area. Jpn J Cancer Res 2001;92(11):1157–65.

97. Wang M, Guo C, Li M. [A case-control study on the dietary risk factors of upper digestive tract cancer]. Zhonghua Liu Xing Bing Xue Za Zhi 1999;20(2):95–7 [in Chinese].

98. Wang Z, Tang L, Sun G, et al. Etiological study of esophageal squamous cell carcinoma in an endemic region: a population-based case control study in Huaian, China. BMC Cancer 2006;6:287.

99. Yang CX, Wang HY, Wang ZM, et al. Risk factors for esophageal cancer: a case-control study in South-western China. Asian Pac J Cancer Prev 2005;6(1):48–53.

100. Hu J, Nyren O, Wolk A, et al. Risk factors for oesophageal cancer in northeast China. Int J Cancer 1994;57(1):38–46.

101. Li JY, Ershow AG, Chen ZJ, et al. A case-control study of cancer of the esophagus and gastric cardia in Linxian. Int J Cancer 1989;43(5):755–61.

102. International Agency for Research on Cancer. Pickled vegetables. IARC Monogr Eval Carcinog Risks Hum 1993;56:83–113.

103. World Cancer Research Fund/American Institute for Cancer Research. Food, nutrition, physical activity, and the prevention of cancer: a global perspective. Washington, DC: AICR; 2007.

104. Freedman ND, Park Y, Subar AF, et al. Fruit and vegetable intake and esophageal cancer in a large prospective cohort study. Int J Cancer 2007;121(12):2753–60.

105. Gonzalez CA, Pera G, Agudo A, et al. Fruit and vegetable intake and the risk of stomach and oesophagus adenocarcinoma in the European Prospective Investigation into Cancer and Nutrition (EPIC-EURGAST). Int J Cancer 2006;118(10):2559–66.

106. Yamaji T, Inoue M, Sasazuki S, et al. Fruit and vegetable consumption and squamous cell carcinoma of the esophagus in Japan: the JPHC study. Int J Cancer 2008;123(8):1935–40.

107. Yang CS, Sun Y, Yang QU, et al. Vitamin A and other deficiencies in Linxian, a high esophageal cancer incidence area in Northern China. J Natl Cancer Inst 1984;73(6):1449–53.

108. Li JY, Taylor PR, Li B, et al. Nutrition intervention trials in Linxian, China: multiple vitamin/mineral supplementation, cancer incidence, and disease-specific mortality among adults with esophageal dysplasia. J Natl Cancer Inst 1993;85(18):1492–8.

109. Blot WJ, Li JY, Taylor PR, et al. Nutrition intervention trials in Linxian, China: supplementation with specific vitamin/mineral combinations, cancer incidence, and disease-specific mortality in the general population. J Natl Cancer Inst 1993;85(18):1483–92.

110. Taylor PR, Qiao YL, Dawsey SM, et al. Total and cancer mortality following supplementation with multi-vitamins and minerals: Post-intervention follow-up of the general population nutrition intervention trial in Linxian, China. Cancer Epidemiol Biomarkers Prev 2004;13(11):1843S.

111. Omenn GS, Goodman G, Thornquist M, et al. Chemoprevention of lung cancer: the beta-Carotene and Retinol Efficacy Trial (CARET) in high-risk smokers and asbestos-exposed workers. IARC Sci Publ 1996;(136):67–85.

112. The ATBC Cancer Prevention Study Group. The effect of vitamin E and beta carotene on the incidence of lung cancer and other cancers in male smokers. The Alpha-Tocopherol, Beta Carotene Cancer Prevention Study Group. N Engl J Med 1994;330(15):1029–35.

113. Bjelakovic G, Nikolova D, Simonetti RG, et al. Antioxidant supplements for prevention of gastrointestinal cancers: a systematic review and meta-analysis. Lancet 2004;364(9441):1219–28.

114. Bjelakovic G, Nikolova D, Gluud LL, et al. Mortality in randomized trials of antioxidant supplements for primary and secondary prevention: systematic review and meta-analysis. JAMA 2007;297(8):842–57.

115. Knekt P, Aromaa A, Maatela J, et al. Serum selenium and subsequent risk of cancer among Finnish men and women. J Natl Cancer Inst 1990;82(10): 864–8.
116. Mark SD, Qiao YL, Dawsey SM, et al. Prospective study of serum selenium levels and incident esophageal and gastric cancers. J Natl Cancer Inst 2000; 92(21):1753–63.
117. Wei WQ, Abnet CC, Qiao YL, et al. Prospective study of serum selenium concentrations and esophageal and gastric cardia cancer, heart disease, stroke, and total death. Am J Clin Nutr 2004;79(1):80–5.
118. Limburg PJ, Wei W, Ahnen DJ, et al. Randomized, placebo-controlled, esophageal squamous cell cancer chemoprevention trial of selenomethionine and celecoxib. Gastroenterology 2005;129(3):863–73.
119. Fong LY, Magee PN. Dietary zinc deficiency enhances esophageal cell proliferation and N-nitrosomethylbenzylamine (NMBA)-induced esophageal tumor incidence in C57BL/6 mouse. Cancer Lett 1999;143(1):63–9.
120. Fong LY, Sivak A, Newberne PM. Zinc deficiency and methylbenzylnitrosamine-induced esophageal cancer in rats. J Natl Cancer Inst 1978;61(1):145–50.
121. Abnet CC, Lai B, Qiao YL, et al. Zinc concentration in esophageal biopsy specimens measured by x-ray fluorescence and esophageal cancer risk. J Natl Cancer Inst 2005;97(4):301–6.
122. Corley DA, Kerlikowske K, Verma R, et al. Protective association of aspirin/ NSAIDs and esophageal cancer: a systematic review and meta-analysis. Gastroenterology 2003;124(1):47–56.
123. Lindblad M, Lagergren J, Garcia Rodriguez LA. Nonsteroidal anti-inflammatory drugs and risk of esophageal and gastric cancer. Cancer Epidemiol Biomarkers Prev 2005;14(2):444–50.
124. Anderson LA, Johnston BT, Watson RG, et al. Nonsteroidal anti-inflammatory drugs and the esophageal inflammation-metaplasia-adenocarcinoma sequence. Cancer Res 2006;66(9):4975–82.
125. Ranka S, Gee JM, Johnson IT, et al. Non-steroidal anti-inflammatory drugs, lower oesophageal sphincter-relaxing drugs and oesophageal cancer. A case-control study. Digestion 2006;74(2):109–15.
126. Fortuny J, Johnson CC, Bohlke K, et al. Use of anti-inflammatory drugs and lower esophageal sphincter-relaxing drugs and risk of esophageal and gastric cancers. Clin Gastroenterol Hepatol 2007;5(10):1154–9.
127. Duan L, Wu AH, Sullivan-Halley J, et al. Nonsteroidal anti-inflammatory drugs and risk of esophageal and gastric adenocarcinomas in Los Angeles County. Cancer Epidemiol Biomarkers Prev 2008;17(1):126–34.
128. Jankowski J, Moayyedi P. Re: Cost-effectiveness of aspirin chemoprevention for Barrett's esophagus. J Natl Cancer Inst 2004;96(11):885–7.
129. Wang HH, Hsieh CC, Antonioli DA. Rising incidence rate of esophageal adenocarcinoma and use of pharmaceutical agents that relax the lower esophageal sphincter (United States). Cancer Causes Control 1994;5(6):573–8.
130. Vaughan TL, Farrow DC, Hansten PD, et al. Risk of esophageal and gastric adenocarcinomas in relation to use of calcium channel blockers, asthma drugs, and other medications that promote gastroesophageal reflux. Cancer Epidemiol Biomarkers Prev 1998;7(9):749–56.
131. Corley DA, Levin TR, Habel LA, et al. Barrett's esophagus and medications that relax the lower esophageal sphincter. Am J Gastroenterol 2006;101(5): 937–44.

132. Lagergren J, Bergstrom R, Adami HO, et al. Association between medications that relax the lower esophageal sphincter and risk for esophageal adenocarcinoma. Ann Intern Med 2000;133(3):165–75.

133. Ye W, Chow WH, Lagergren J, et al. Risk of adenocarcinomas of the oesophagus and gastric cardia in patients hospitalized for asthma. Br J Cancer 2001;85(9):1317–21.

134. Foster AB, Jarman M, Manson D, et al. Structure and reactivity of nitrosocimetidine. Cancer Lett 1980;9(1):47–52.

135. Chow WH, Finkle WD, McLaughlin JK, et al. The relation of gastroesophageal reflux disease and its treatment to adenocarcinomas of the esophagus and gastric cardia. JAMA 1995;274(6):474–7.

136. Colin-Jones DG, Langman MJ, Lawson DH, et al. Post-cimetidine surveillance for up to ten years: incidence of carcinoma of the stomach and oesophagus. QJM 1991;78(285):13–9.

137. Farrow DC, Vaughan TL, Sweeney C, et al. Gastroesophageal reflux disease, use of H2 receptor antagonists, and risk of esophageal and gastric cancer. Cancer Causes Control 2000;11(3):231–8.

138. Garcia Rodriguez LA, Lagergren J, Lindblad M. Gastric acid suppression and risk of oesophageal and gastric adenocarcinoma: a nested case control study in the UK. Gut 2006;55(11):1538–44.

139. Suleiman UL, Harrison M, Britton A, et al. H2-receptor antagonists may increase the risk of cardio-oesophageal adenocarcinoma: a case-control study. Eur J Cancer Prev 2000;9(3):185–91.

140. Suerbaum S, Michetti P. *Helicobacter pylori* infection. N Engl J Med 2002; 347(15):1175–86.

141. Islami F, Kamangar F. *Helicobacter pylori* and esophageal cancer risk—a meta-analysis. Cancer Prev Res (Phila Pa) 2008;1(5):329–38.

142. Rokkas T, Pistiolas D, Sechopoulos P, et al. Relationship between *Helicobacter pylori* infection and esophageal neoplasia: a meta-analysis. Clin Gastroenterol Hepatol 2007;5(12):1413–7.

143. Zhuo X, Zhang Y, Wang Y, et al. *Helicobacter pylori* infection and oesophageal cancer risk: association studies via evidence-based meta-analyses. Clin Oncol (R Coll Radiol) 2008;20(10):757–62.

144. Chow WH, Blaser MJ, Blot WJ, et al. An inverse relation between cagA+ strains of *Helicobacter pylori* infection and risk of esophageal and gastric cardia adenocarcinoma. Cancer Res 1998;58(4):588–90.

145. Wren AM, Bloom SR. Gut hormones and appetite control. Gastroenterology 2007;132(6):2116–30.

146. Blaser MJ. Who are we? Indigenous microbes and the ecology of human diseases. EMBO Rep 2006;7(10):956–60.

147. Chen Y, Blaser MJ. *Helicobacter pylori* colonization is inversely associated with childhood asthma. J Infect Dis 2008;198(4):553–60.

148. Sarker SA, Nahar S, Rahman M, et al. High prevalence of cagA and vacA seropositivity in asymptomatic Bangladeshi children with *Helicobacter pylori* infection. Acta Paediatr 2004;93(11):1432–6.

149. El Omar EM, Rabkin CS, Gammon MD, et al. Increased risk of noncardia gastric cancer associated with proinflammatory cytokine gene polymorphisms. Gastroenterology 2003;124(5):1193–201.

150. Kamangar F, Qiao YL, Blaser MJ, et al. *Helicobacter pylori* and oesophageal and gastric cancers in a prospective study in China. Br J Cancer 2007;96(1):172–6.

151. Wu DC, Wu IC, Lee JM, et al. *Helicobacter pylori* infection: a protective factor for esophageal squamous cell carcinoma in a Taiwanese population. Am J Gastroenterol 2005;100(3):588–93.
152. Munoz N, Bosch FX, de Sanjose S, et al. Epidemiologic classification of human papillomavirus types associated with cervical cancer. N Engl J Med 2003; 348(6):518–27.
153. International Agency for Research on Cancer. Human papillomaviruses. IARC Monogr Eval Carcinog Risks Hum 2007;90:1–636.
154. Gillison ML, Shah KV. Chapter 9: role of mucosal human papillomavirus in nongenital cancers. J Natl Cancer Inst Monographs 2003;(31):57–65.
155. Syrjanen K, Pyrhonen S, Aukee S, et al. Squamous cell papilloma of the esophagus: a tumour probably caused by human papilloma virus (HPV). Diagn Histopathol 1982;5(4):291–6.
156. Syrjanen KJ. HPV infections and oesophageal cancer. J Clin Pathol 2002;55(10): 721–8.
157. Benamouzig R, Jullian E, Chang F, et al. Absence of human papillomavirus DNA detected by polymerase chain reaction in French patients with esophageal carcinoma. Gastroenterology 1995;109(6):1876–81.
158. Koh JS, Lee SS, Baek HJ, et al. No association of high-risk human papillomavirus with esophageal squamous cell carcinomas among Koreans, as determined by polymerase chain reaction. Dis Esophagus 2008;21(2):114–7.
159. Kok TC, Nooter K, Tjong AHS, et al. No evidence of known types of human papillomavirus in squamous cell cancer of the oesophagus in a low-risk area. Rotterdam Oesophageal Tumour Study Group. Eur J Cancer 1997;33(11):1865–8.
160. Poljak M, Cerar A, Seme K. Human papillomavirus infection in esophageal carcinomas: a study of 121 lesions using multiple broad-spectrum polymerase chain reactions and literature review. Hum Pathol 1998;29(3):266–71.
161. Saegusa M, Hashimura M, Takano Y, et al. Absence of human papillomavirus genomic sequences detected by the polymerase chain reaction in oesophageal and gastric carcinomas in Japan. Mol Pathol 1997;50(2):101–4.
162. Talamini G, Capelli P, Zamboni G, et al. Alcohol, smoking and papillomavirus infection as risk factors for esophageal squamous-cell papilloma and esophageal squamous-cell carcinoma in Italy. Int J Cancer 2000;86(6):874–8.
163. White RE, Mungatana C, Mutuma G, et al. Absence of human papillomavirus in esophageal carcinomas from southwestern Kenya. Dis Esophagus 2005;18(1): 28–30.
164. Yao PF, Li GC, Li J, et al. Evidence of human papilloma virus infection and its epidemiology in esophageal squamous cell carcinoma. World J Gastroenterol 2006;12(9):1352–5.
165. Dillner J, Knekt P, Schiller JT, et al. Prospective seroepidemiological evidence that human papillomavirus type 16 infection is a risk factor for oesophageal squamous cell carcinoma. BMJ 1995;311(7016):1346.
166. Bjorge T, Hakulinen T, Engeland A, et al. A prospective, seroepidemiological study of the role of human papillomavirus in esophageal cancer in Norway. Cancer Res 1997;57(18):3989–92.
167. Han C, Qiao G, Hubbert NL, et al. Serologic association between human papillomavirus type 16 infection and esophageal cancer in Shaanxi Province, China. J Natl Cancer Inst 1996;88(20):1467–71.
168. Lagergren J, Wang Z, Bergstrom R, et al. Human papillomavirus infection and esophageal cancer: a nationwide seroepidemiologic case-control study in Sweden. J Natl Cancer Inst 1999;91(2):156–62.

169. van Doornum GJ, Korse CM, Buning-Kager JC, et al. Reactivity to human papillomavirus type 16 L1 virus-like particles in sera from patients with genital cancer and patients with carcinomas at five different extragenital sites. Br J Cancer 2003;88(7):1095–100.

170. Kamangar F, Qiao YL, Schiller JT, et al. Human papillomavirus serology and the risk of esophageal and gastric cancers: results from a cohort in a high-risk region in China. Int J Cancer 2006;119(3):579–84.

171. Kazerouni N, Sinha R, Hsu CH, et al. Analysis of 200 food items for benzo[a]pyrene and estimation of its intake in an epidemiologic study. Food Chem Toxicol 2001;39(5):423–36.

172. Chang KF, Fang GC, Chen JC, et al. Atmospheric polycyclic aromatic hydrocarbons (PAHs) in Asia: a review from 1999 to 2004. Environ Pollut 2006;142(3):388–96.

173. Mastrangelo G, Fadda E, Marzia V. Polycyclic aromatic hydrocarbons and cancer in man. Environ Health Perspect 1996;104(11):1166–70.

174. Pott P. Chirurgical observations. Natl Cancer Inst Monogr 1963;10:7.

175. Luch A. Nature and nurture—lessons from chemical carcinogenesis. Nat Rev Cancer 2005;5(2):113–25.

176. Boffetta P, Jourenkova N, Gustavsson P. Cancer risk from occupational and environmental exposure to polycyclic aromatic hydrocarbons. Cancer Causes Control 1997;8(3):444–72.

177. Roth MJ, Guo-Qing W, Lewin KJ, et al. Histopathologic changes seen in esophagectomy specimens from the high-risk region of Linxian, China: potential clues to an etiologic exposure? Hum Pathol 1998;29(11):1294–8.

178. Roth MJ, Strickland KL, Wang GQ, et al. High levels of carcinogenic polycyclic aromatic hydrocarbons present within food from Linxian, China may contribute to that region's high incidence of oesophageal cancer. Eur J Cancer 1998;34(5): 757–8.

179. Roth M, Qiao Y, Rothman N, et al. High urine 1-hydroxypyrene glucoronide concentration in Linxian, China, an area of high risk for squamous oesophageal cancer. Biomarkers 2001;6(5):381–6.

180. Kamangar F, Strickland PT, Pourshams A, et al. High exposure to polycyclic aromatic hydrocarbons may contribute to high risk of esophageal cancer in northeastern Iran. Anticancer Res 2005;25(1B):425–8.

181. Strickland P, Kang D, Sithisarankul P. Polycyclic aromatic hydrocarbon metabolites in urine as biomarkers of exposure and effect. Environ Health Perspect 1996;104(Suppl 5):927–32.

182. Lewtas J, Walsh D, Williams R, et al. Air pollution exposure-DNA adduct dosimetry in humans and rodents: evidence for non-linearity at high doses. Mutat Res 1997;378(1–2):51–63.

183. van Schooten FJ, Godschalk RW, Breedijk A, et al. 32P-postlabelling of aromatic DNA adducts in white blood cells and alveolar macrophages of smokers: saturation at high exposures. Mutat Res 1997;378(1–2):65–75.

184. Fong LY, Lau KM, Huebner K, et al. Induction of esophageal tumors in zinc-deficient rats by single low doses of N-nitrosomethylbenzylamine (NMBA): analysis of cell proliferation, and mutations in H-ras and p53 genes. Carcinogenesis 1997;18(8):1477–84.

185. Lijinsky W, Kovatch RM. Induction of liver tumors in rats by nitrosodiethanolamine at low doses. Carcinogenesis 1985;6(12):1679–81.

186. Ivankovic S, Seibel J, Komitowski D, et al. Caffeine-derived N-nitroso compounds. V. Carcinogenicity of mononitrosocaffeidine and dinitrosocaffeidine in bd-ix rats. Carcinogenesis 1998;19(5):933–7.

187. Preussmann R, Habs M, Habs H, et al. Fluoro-substituted N-nitrosamines. 6. carcinogenicity of N-nitroso-(2,2,2-trifluoroethyl)-ethylamine in rats. Carcinogenesis 1983;4(6):755–7.

188. Bartsch H, Spiegelhalder B. Environmental exposure to N-nitroso compounds (NNOC) and precursors: an overview. Eur J Cancer Prev 1996;5(Suppl 1):11–7.

189. Tricker AR. N-nitroso compounds and man: sources of exposure, endogenous formation and occurrence in body fluids. Eur J Cancer Prev 1997;6(3):226–68.

190. Forman D. Dietary exposure to N-nitroso compounds and the risk of human cancer. Cancer Surv 1987;6(4):719–38.

191. Mirvish SS. Role of N-nitroso compounds (NOC) and N-nitrosation in etiology of gastric, esophageal, nasopharyngeal and bladder cancer and contribution to cancer of known exposures to NOC. Cancer Lett 1995;93(1):17–48.

192. Mirvish SS. The etiology of gastric cancer. Intragastric nitrosamide formation and other theories. J Natl Cancer Inst 1983;71(3):629–47.

193. Abnet CC, Qiao YL, Mark SD, et al. Prospective study of tooth loss and incident esophageal and gastric cancers in China. Cancer Causes Control 2001;12(9):847–54.

194. Abnet CC, Kamangar F, Dawsey SM, et al. Tooth loss is associated with increased risk of gastric non-cardia adenocarcinoma in a cohort of Finnish smokers. Scand J Gastroenterol 2005;40(6):681–7.

195. Jakszyn P, Gonzalez CA. Nitrosamine and related food intake and gastric and oesophageal cancer risk: a systematic review of the epidemiological evidence. World J Gastroenterol 2006;12(27):4296–303.

196. Yokoyama A, Omori T. Genetic polymorphisms of alcohol and aldehyde dehydrogenases and risk for esophageal and head and neck cancers. Alcohol 2005;35(3):175–85.

197. International Agency for Research on Cancer. Acetaldehyde. IARC Monogr Eval Carcinog Risks Hum 1999;(71 Pt 2):319–35.

198. Salaspuro M. Interrelationship between alcohol, smoking, acetaldehyde and cancer. Novartis Found Symp 2007;285:80–9.

199. Gelderblom WC, Kriek NP, Marasas WF, et al. Toxicity and carcinogenicity of the *Fusarium moniliforme* metabolite, fumonisin B1, in rats. Carcinogenesis 1991; 12(7):1247–51.

200. Howard PC, Eppley RM, Stack ME, et al. Fumonisin b1 carcinogenicity in a two-year feeding study using F344 rats and B6C3F1 mice. Environ Health Perspect 2001;109(Suppl 2):277–82.

201. Marasas WF, van Rensburg SJ, Mirocha CJ. Incidence of *Fusarium* species and the mycotoxins, deoxynivalenol and zearalenone, in corn produced in esophageal cancer areas in Transkei. J Agric Food Chem 1979;27(5):1108–12.

202. Shephard GS, Marasas WF, Leggott NL, et al. Natural occurrence of fumonisins in corn from Iran. J Agric Food Chem 2000;48(5):1860–4.

203. Chu FS, Li GY. Simultaneous occurrence of fumonisin B1 and other mycotoxins in moldy corn collected from the People's Republic of China in regions with high incidences of esophageal cancer. Appl Environ Microbiol 1994;60(3):847–52.

204. Abnet CC, Borkowf CB, Qiao YL, et al. Sphingolipids as biomarkers of fumonisin exposure and risk of esophageal squamous cell carcinoma in china. Cancer Causes Control 2001;12(9):821–8.

205. Lagergren J, Bergstrom R, Lindgren A, et al. Symptomatic gastroesophageal reflux as a risk factor for esophageal adenocarcinoma. N Engl J Med 1999; 340(11):825–31.

206. Wu AH, Tseng CC, Bernstein L. Hiatal hernia, reflux symptoms, body size, and risk of esophageal and gastric adenocarcinoma. Cancer 2003;98(5):940–8.

207. Lieberman DA, Oehlke M, Helfand M. Risk factors for Barrett's esophagus in community-based practice. GORGE consortium. Gastroenterology Outcomes Research Group in Endoscopy. Am J Gastroenterol 1997;92(8):1293–7.
208. Hampel H, Abraham NS, El-Serag HB. Meta-analysis: obesity and the risk for gastroesophageal reflux disease and its complications. Ann Intern Med 2005; 143(3):199–211.
209. Kubo A, Corley DA. Body mass index and adenocarcinomas of the esophagus or gastric cardia: a systematic review and meta-analysis. Cancer Epidemiol Biomarkers Prev 2006;15(5):872–8.
210. Abnet CC, Freedman ND, Hollenbeck AR, et al. A prospective study of BMI and risk of oesophageal and gastric adenocarcinoma. Eur J Cancer 2008;44(3): 465–71.
211. Corley DA, Kubo A, Zhao W. Abdominal obesity and the risk of esophageal and gastric cardia carcinomas. Cancer Epidemiol Biomarkers Prev 2008;17(2): 352–8.
212. Corley DA. Obesity and the rising incidence of oesophageal and gastric adeno-carcinoma: what is the link? Gut 2007;56(11):1493–4.
213. Corley DA, Kubo A. Body mass index and gastroesophageal reflux disease: a systematic review and meta-analysis. Am J Gastroenterol 2006;101(11):2619–28.
214. Edelstein ZR, Farrow DC, Bronner MP, et al. Central adiposity and risk of Barrett's esophagus. Gastroenterology 2007;133(2):403–11.
215. Corley DA, Kubo A, Levin TR, et al. Abdominal obesity and body mass index as risk factors for Barrett's esophagus. Gastroenterology 2007;133(1):34–41.
216. Weston AP, Sharma P, Mathur S, et al. Risk stratification of Barrett's esophagus: updated prospective multivariate analysis. Am J Gastroenterol 2004;99(9): 1657–66.
217. Avidan B, Sonnenberg A, Schnell TG, et al. Hiatal hernia size, Barrett's length, and severity of acid reflux are all risk factors for esophageal adenocarcinoma. Am J Gastroenterol 2002;97(8):1930–6.
218. Leeuwenburgh I, Haringsma J, Van DH, et al. Long-term risk of oesophagitis, Barrett's oesophagus and oesophageal cancer in achalasia patients. Scand J Gastroenterol Suppl 2006;(243):7–10.
219. Carter R, Brewer LA III. Achalasia and esophageal carcinoma. Studies in early diagnosis for improved surgical management. Am J Surg 1975;130(2):114–20.
220. Wychulis AR, Woolam GL, Andersen HA, et al. Achalasia and carcinoma of the esophagus. JAMA 1971;215(10):1638–41.
221. Meijssen MA, Tilanus HW, van BM, et al. Achalasia complicated by oesophageal squamous cell carcinoma: a prospective study in 195 patients. Gut 1992;33(2): 155–8.
222. Streitz JM Jr, Ellis FH Jr, Gibb SP, et al. Achalasia and squamous cell carcinoma of the esophagus: analysis of 241 patients. Ann Thorac Surg 1995;59(6): 1604–9.
223. Zendehdel K, Nyren O, Edberg A, et al. Risk of esophageal adenocarcinoma in achalasia patients, a retrospective cohort study in Sweden. Am J Gastroenterol, in press.
224. Joske RA, Benedict EB. The role of benign esophageal obstruction in the devel-opment of carcinoma of the esophagus. Gastroenterology 1959;36(6):749–55.
225. Correa P. A human model of gastric carcinogenesis. Cancer Res 1988;48(13): 3554–60.
226. Hsing AW, Hansson LE, McLaughlin JK, et al. Pernicious anemia and subse-quent cancer. A population-based cohort study. Cancer 1993;71(3):745–50.

227. Ye W, Nyren O. Risk of cancers of the oesophagus and stomach by histology or subsite in patients hospitalised for pernicious anaemia. Gut 2003;52(7): 938–41.

228. Ley C, Mohar A, Guarner J, et al. Screening markers for chronic atrophic gastritis in Chiapas, Mexico. Cancer Epidemiol Biomarkers Prev 2001;10(2):107–12.

229. Samloff IM, Varis K, Ihamaki T, et al. Relationships among serum pepsinogen I, serum pepsinogen II, and gastric mucosal histology. A study in relatives of patients with pernicious anemia. Gastroenterology 1982;83(1 Pt 2):204–9.

230. Ye W, Held M, Lagergren J, et al. *Helicobacter pylori* infection and gastric atrophy: risk of adenocarcinoma and squamous-cell carcinoma of the esophagus and adenocarcinoma of the gastric cardia. J Natl Cancer Inst 2004; 96(5):388–96.

231. Iijima K, Koike T, Abe Y, et al. Extensive gastric atrophy: an increased risk factor for superficial esophageal squamous cell carcinoma in Japan. Am J Gastroenterol 2007;102(8):1603–9.

232. Kamangar F, Diaw L, Wei WQ, et al. Serum pepsinogens and risk of esophageal squamous dysplasia. Int J Cancer 2008;124:456–60.

233. de Vries AC, Capelle LG, Looman CWN, et al. Increased risk of esophageal squamous cell carcinoma in patients with gastric atrophy: independent of the severity of atrophic changes. Int J Cancer, in press.

234. Correa P. Human gastric carcinogenesis: a multistep and multifactorial process—first American Cancer Society Award Lecture on Cancer Epidemiology and Prevention. Cancer Res 1992;52(24):6735–40.

235. Abnet CC, Qiao YL, Dawsey SM, et al. Tooth loss is associated with increased risk of total death and death from upper gastrointestinal cancer, heart disease, and stroke in a Chinese population-based cohort. Int J Epidemiol 2005;34(2): 467–74.

236. Guha N, Boffetta P, Wunsch F, et al. Oral health and risk of squamous cell carcinoma of the head and neck and esophagus: results of two multicentric case-control studies. Am J Epidemiol 2007;166(10):1159–73.

237. Hiraki A, Matsuo K, Suzuki T, et al. Teeth loss and risk of cancer at 14 common sites in Japanese. Cancer Epidemiol Biomarkers Prev 2008;17(5):1222–7.

238. Abnet CC, Kamangar F, Islami F, et al. Tooth loss and lack of regular oral hygiene are associated with higher risk of esophageal squamous cell carcinoma in a case-control study conducted in Golestan Province, Iran. Cancer Epidemiol Biomarkers Prev 2008;17(11):3062–8.

239. Sepehr A, Kamangar F, Fahimi S, et al. Poor oral health as a risk factor for esophageal squamous dysplasia in northeastern Iran. Anticancer Res 2005; 25(1B):543–6.

240. Wei WQ, Abnet CC, Lu N, et al. Risk factors for oesophageal squamous dysplasia in adult inhabitants of a high risk region of China. Gut 2005;54(6): 759–63.

241. Gustavsson P, Evanoff B, Hogstedt C. Increased risk of esophageal cancer among workers exposed to combustion products. Arch Environ Health 1993; 48(4):243–5.

242. Hein MJ, Stayner LT, Lehman E, et al. Follow-up study of chrysotile textile workers: cohort mortality and exposure-response. Occup Environ Med 2007; 64(9):616–25.

243. Jansson C, Johansson AL, Bergdahl IA, et al. Occupational exposures and risk of esophageal and gastric cardia cancers among male Swedish construction workers. Cancer Causes Control 2005;16(6):755–64.

244. Santibanez M, Vioque J, Alguacil J, et al. Occupational exposures and risk of oesophageal cancer by historical type: a case control study in eastern Spain. Occup Environ Med 2008;65:774–81.

245. Wernli KJ, Fitzgibbons ED, Ray RM, et al. Occupational risk factors for esophageal and stomach cancers among female textile workers in Shanghai, China. Am J Epidemiol 2006;163(8):717–25.

246. Cucino C, Sonnenberg A. Occupational mortality from squamous cell carcinoma of the esophagus in the United States during 1991–1996. Dig Dis Sci 2002; 47(3):568–72.

247. Fillmore CM, Petralia SA, Dosemeci M. Cancer mortality in women with probable exposure to silica: a death certificate study in 24 states of the U.S. Am J Ind Med 1999;36(1):122–8.

248. Pan G, Takahashi K, Feng Y, et al. Nested case-control study of esophageal cancer in relation to occupational exposure to silica and other dusts. Am J Ind Med 1999;35(3):272–80.

249. Yu IT, Tse LA, Wong TW, et al. Further evidence for a link between silica dust and esophageal cancer. Int J Cancer 2005;114(3):479–83.

250. Kang SK, Burnett CA, Freund E, et al. Gastrointestinal cancer mortality of workers in occupations with high asbestos exposures. Am J Ind Med 1997; 31(6):713–8.

251. International Agency for Research on Cancer. Silica, some silicates, coal dust and para-aramid fibrils. IARC Monogr Eval Carcinog Risks Hum 1997;68:1–475.

252. International Agency for Research on Cancer. Asbestos. IARC Monogr Eval Carcinog Risk Chem Man 1977;14:1–106.

253. Ahmed WU, Qureshi H, Alam E, et al. Oesophageal carcinoma in Karachi. J Pak Med Assoc 1992;42(6):133–5.

254. Bosetti C, Franceschi S, Negri E, et al. Changing socioeconomic correlates for cancers of the upper digestive tract. Ann Oncol 2001;12(3):327–30.

255. De Jong UW, Breslow N, Hong JG, et al. Aetiological factors in oesophageal cancer in Singapore Chinese. Int J Cancer 1974;13(3):291–303.

256. Jansson C, Johansson AL, Nyren O, et al. Socioeconomic factors and risk of esophageal adenocarcinoma: a nationwide Swedish case-control study. Cancer Epidemiol Biomarkers Prev 2005;14(7):1754–61.

257. Nagel G, Linseisen J, Boshuizen HC, et al. Socioeconomic position and the risk of gastric and oesophageal cancer in the European Prospective Investigation into Cancer and Nutrition (EPIC-EURGAST). Int J Epidemiol 2007;36(1):66–76.

258. Shai D. Cancer mortality, ethnicity, and socioeconomic status: two New York City groups. Public Health Rep 1986;101(5):547–52.

259. Vizcaino AP, Parkin DM, Skinner ME. Risk factors associated with oesophageal cancer in Bulawayo, Zimbabwe. Br J Cancer 1995;72(3):769–73.

260. Weiderpass E, Pukkala E. Time trends in socioeconomic differences in incidence rates of cancers of gastro-intestinal tract in Finland. BMC Gastroenterol 2006;6:41.

261. Brewster DH, Fraser LA, McKinney PA, et al. Socioeconomic status and risk of adenocarcinoma of the oesophagus and cancer of the gastric cardia in Scotland. Br J Cancer 2000;83(3):387–90.

Screening, Surveillance, and Prevention for Esophageal Cancer

Yutaka Tomizawa, MD, Kenneth K. Wang, MD*

KEYWORDS

- Adenocarcinoma • Barrett's • Endoscopy
- Esophageal • Squamous

Strategies to screen, survey, and prevent esophageal cancer must take into account the changing epidemiology of the disease. Esophageal cancer is relatively uncommon; however, it is the second leading cancer in terms of its ever-increasing incidence. When it occurs, esophageal cancer has one of the highest mortality rates in the United States. In 2008, an estimated 16,470 new patients were diagnosed with esophageal cancer and 14,280 individuals died of this disease.[1] Recent reports show esophageal adenocarcinoma incidence rates rose from 1975 through 2004 among white men and women in all stages and age groups. The incidence of adenocarcinoma among white men increased 463%, from 1.01 per 100,000 person-years in 1975–1979 to 5.69 per 100,000 person-years in 2000–2004. A similar rapid increase was also apparent among white women, with an increased incidence of 335% from 0.17 per 100,000 person-years to 0.74 per 100,000 person-years.[2] This increase was not found in earlier reports because of the rarity of EAC among women. Squamous cell carcinoma of the esophagus is now less common than adenocarcinoma in the United States and is thought to be due to decreased consumption of alcohol and tobacco. It is clear that to affect the increasing rate of esophageal cancer and to improve its prognosis, it is necessary to develop new strategies of screening, surveillance, and prevention.

SQUAMOUS CELL CARCINOMA

In contrast to the situation in the United States, squamous cell carcinoma is the most common type of esophageal cancer worldwide, where it remains a significant health

This article is supported by NIH grants R01CA111603-01A1, R01CA097048, and R21CA122426-01.

Barrett's Esophagus Unit, Alfred Main, Gastroenterology Diagnostic Unit, St. Mary's Hospital, 200 2nd Street SW, Rochester, MN 55905, USA

* Corresponding author. Barrett's Esophagus Unit, Alfred Main, Gastroenterology Diagnostic Unit, St. Mary's Hospital, 200 2nd Street SW, Rochester, MN 55905.

E-mail address: wang.kenneth@mayo.edu (K.K. Wang).

care burden, particularly in Asian countries, which have a high incidence of squamous cell carcinoma.[3] In the United States, squamous cell carcinoma is the most common type of esophageal cancer in African American and Hispanic males. Alcohol consumption, smoking, consumption of food and water rich in nitrates and nitrosamines, and specific genetic factors have all been reported as risk factors for cancer development. In addition, Plummer-Vinson syndrome, achalasia, and chronic strictures resulting from acid or lye ingestion have all been implicated as predisposing factors.[4] Although some case-control studies to evaluate familial aggregation were conducted in China, a region where the incidence of squamous cell carcinoma is high, it remains unclear whether squamous cell carcinoma is heritable.[5] Tylosis, a genetic defect in the 17q25 region characterized by hyperkeratosis of the palms and soles is associated with high risk of squamous cell carcinoma by the age of 65 years.[6] Based on experimental evidence, squamous cell carcinoma is believed to develop via progression through a premalignant dysplastic phase before development of carcinoma. Although there are many studies regarding molecular pathogenesis (p53, Rb, and p16 are common alterations) of squamous dysplasia and squamous cell carcinoma, it remains unclear if unique signaling pathways exist in these conditions. Known biologic processes such as methylation have been shown to play a role in the pathogenesis of both squamous and adenocarcinoma.

BARRETT'S ESOPHAGUS AND ESOPHAGEAL ADENOCARCINOMA

The known risk factors for esophageal adenocarcinoma (EAC) are chronic gastroesophageal reflux disease (GERD) and Barrett's esophagus (BE).[7] Persons with recurring symptoms of reflux have an eightfold increase in the risk of EAC.[8] Among patients with BE, the annual rate of neoplastic transformation is reported as approximately 0.5%, although this estimate is based on compiled series with relatively short follow-up times.[9] It seems unlikely that someone diagnosed with BE at age 50 would have a 10% cumulative risk of cancer by age 70 based on current information. Barrett's is a condition in which normal squamous epithelium of the esophagus is replaced by metaplastic columnar mucosa. This phenomenon is a complication of esophageal mucosal damage caused by GERD.[10] It is thought that histologic evidence of intestinal metaplasia is required before BE can progress sequentially from no dysplasia to low-grade dysplasia, then to high-grade dysplasia, and eventually to adenocarcinoma. It should be noted that this theory is controversial due to several reports of progression to adenocarcinoma without precursor lesions of intestinalized epithelium with goblet cells. However, other markers of intestinal metaplasia, such as cytokeratin profiles or expression of intestinal transcription factors such as CDX2, are usually found in non-goblet cells containing intestinalized mucosa.

Progression of BE to cancer is felt to be a relatively slow process, although there is an increase in cancer rates due to the difficulty in detecting cancers early with random biopsies.[11] Most cancers within BE are found early after diagnosis and the rates of progression after the first year of diagnosis are significantly decreased. Although BE is recognized as a premalignant condition, it does not produce any symptoms itself. Some have thought that the incidence of clinically diagnosed BE has increased as a result of the increased use of endoscopy, others have found that this is not the case.[12] It is generally accepted that Barrett's esophagus is increasing.

Early diagnosis of BE is critical because metastasis is common with the evolution to carcinoma. The lymphatic supply of the esophagus reaches the lamina propria, lymph node metastasis can occur even in early-stage disease. The prognosis of adenocarcinoma is highly dependent on the stage of the disease. Early neoplastic lesions generally have an excellent prognosis, but the prognosis of most advanced lesions is dismal. The goal of screening is to detect patients with BE, the precursor lesion. The goal of surveillance is to diagnose early stages of EAC in patients with known BE and to intervene so as to prevent progression to fatal cancer.[11]

SCREENING

Screening for squamous cell carcinoma in the general population in the United States is not recommended due to the low incidence of this type of esophageal cancer[13] and should only be considered for specific subgroups with known risk factors. Patients with oral and oropharyngeal cancer are well known to have high risk of concomitant esophageal squamous cell carcinoma[14] and should be screened for this disease. Screening should also be considered for patients with tylosis. A screening program is promoted by the concept that detection of early neoplasia can lead to an improved outcome. Recent guidelines state that screening for BE still remains controversial because of the lack of documented impact on mortality from adenocarcinoma of the esophagus.[15] Who, when, how and how often to screen for the presence of BE and adenocarcinoma are frequently raised controversies. Because patients are often asymptomatic, it is difficult to identify the entire at-risk group. It is left to the discretion of the physician to determine if screening is necessary given the health of the patient and the likelihood of early disease. Patients with the higher likelihood of BE are generally older white males with chronic reflux symptoms. It would therefore seem rational to screen those high-risk patients; however, such a strategy works only if those high-risk patients comprise a majority of patients who develop cancer. Although several studies showed reflux symptoms are strongly associated with cancer risk, one report demonstrated that about 40% of subjects with adenocarcinoma reported no antecedent symptoms of reflux.[8] These data indicate a substantial number of patients develop adenocarcinoma without identifiable symptoms of GERD. Presumably such a large number of people would be missed by a screening strategy that emphasized symptoms. However, to screen those patients who lack reflux symptoms but have BE would entail screening the entire population over a specific age. Multiple other risk factors for BE have been identified and several studies attempted to predict the presence of BE.[16,17] Age greater than 40, long duration of GERD symptoms, male gender and hiatus hernia[18] have been suggested as significant risk factors, and at this time the only symptom consistently identified in different studies is heartburn.

Standard endoscopy with biopsy is the most reliable means of establishing a diagnosis of BE. However, it has several limitations as a screening tool, including its low negative predictive value, risk, unpleasant experience, and cost. High negative predictive value is necessary for endoscopy to be a valid screening tool. The negative predictive value of an endoscopy seems to be low and does not meet the level needed for a valid screening method. In one large population-based study which analyzed a total of 589 patients with esophageal or gastric cardia adenocarcinoma, BE was diagnosed in 135 of 589 adenocarcinoma patients and only 23 out of 64 patients who had endoscopy performed more than 6 months before their diagnosis of cancer were identified to have BE.[19] This indicates far fewer patients with adenocarcinoma have an endoscopically recognizable Barrett's segment than we traditionally expect. A systematic review of the prevalence of BE in adenocarcinoma undergoing resection showed only 4.7% of patients undergoing resection reported a prior diagnosis of BE.[20]

Complications of endoscopy related to diagnostic evaluations are rare but can occur especially for elderly patients. It is estimated cardiopulmonary complications related to sedation and analgesia are the most common type of problems seen with diagnostic endoscopy. Though these complications are generally minor changes in vital signs in most of the cases, myocardial infarction, respiratory depression, and shock can occur, albeit rarely.[21]

Unsedated small caliber upper endoscopy is feasible, tolerable, and accurate compared with conventional sedated endoscopy.[22] Unsedated endoscopy has the potential advantage of decreasing sedation-related complications and can be performed as an outpatient procedure in any setting, which could reduce health care costs. However, in this study only five cases of BE were evaluated and limited information is available on unsedated endoscopy in the diagnosis of BE as a screening test. It is yet unknown whether an unsedated procedure will meet with patient acceptance in the United States, given the cultural preference for sedation. Another study in which a smaller caliber scope was used for unsedated patients showed that the diagnostic accuracy of unsedated small-caliber endoscopy was below the acceptable range for esophageal disease, especially for detecting BE.[23] It seems the thinner the caliber is, the more acceptant the modality is for patients; however, as the caliber of the endoscope decreases, the diagnostic accuracy also decreases. Transnasal endoscopy is also attractive as a screening modality because it can be applied as an unsedated technique. This diagnostic modality was assessed its feasibility for surveillance of patients with BE and its relatively high accuracy proved its potential as a screening modality.[24] However, acceptance among referring physicians and the public is also a limiting factor. Despite transnasal endoscopy actually being better tolerated, the public perception is that of greater discomfort. Esophageal capsule endoscopy is a new technique that has the potential to provide a noninvasive diagnosis of suspected BE. The Pillcam ESO video capsule (Given, Yoqneam, Israel) is a dual-camera wireless capsule endoscope developed specifically for esophageal visualization. A pilot feasibility study with 17 subjects showed its safety and capability of imaging the esophagus clearly.[25] A recently published study assessed the accuracy of capsule endoscopy for the diagnosis of BE.[26] In a prospective blinded study of 90 subjects with BE who underwent capsule endoscopy followed by upper endoscopy, capsule endoscopy had only moderate sensitivity and specificity (67% and 84%, respectively) for identification of BE, and positive and negative predictive value were 22% and 98%, respectively. Although this screening method is more acceptable for patients due to convenience and safety, improvement in its diagnostic accuracy is needed to replace upper endoscopy as a standard screening modality.

Barrett's esophagus is frequently suspected at endoscopy, especially for patients with GERD symptoms; however, correctly diagnosing BE can be problematic. One study was conducted to evaluate the ability of the endoscopist to predict the presence of BE at index endoscopy.[27] In the study, endoscopists' interpretations were analyzed with histologic specimens from areas thought to contain BE and positive predictive value was only 34%. Endoscopic detection is difficult because it is based on subtle mucosal changes, and for this reason accurate detection is more difficult in a short segment lesion. New imaging modalities have been developed as adjuncts to white light endoscopy for better visualization of the mucosal changes. Narrow-band imaging is easy to use and allows clear visualization of the mucosal pit patterns and capillary patterns. It showed that the combined recognition of mucosal patterns and capillary patterns improved the diagnostic value for detecting intestinal metaplasia.[28] The same phenomena were reported in other studies and most groups created their own classification of mucosal or vascular patterns correlating to histologic findings. Standardization of the patterns and randomized studies comparing narrow-band imaging with standard endoscopy with biopsy would help to determine an actual clinical impact. Autofluorescence imaging is another promising imaging modality that can differentiate tissue types based on differences in autofluorescence emission. A new endoscopic system has been developed that incorporates high-resolution endoscopy, autofluorescence imaging, and narrow-band imaging in one system. Another recently published international multicenter feasibility study showed that the addition of high-resolution autofluorescence imaging increased the detection of both the number of patients and the number of lesions in patients with BE and the false-positive rate was reduced after detailed inspection with narrow-band imaging.[29] To evaluate its true value as an imaging modality, randomized comparison studies are needed. Although sensitivity and specificity can be assessed from cohort studies, the actual clinical efficacy of these models depends on their acceptability in the community. Currently, there are no validated alternative techniques to screen for BE and consensus is that standard endoscopy with biopsy is the most reliable means of establishing a diagnosis of BE.

In an effort to determine when and how often to screen for BE, several cost-effectiveness models have been produced. One study assessed the cost-effectiveness of performing an initial endoscopic screening of patients with GERD to rule out high-grade dysplasia of BE.[30] Under favorable conditions, this one-time screening endoscopy of all patients with reflux symptoms to prevent death from EAC could be cost-effective compared with no screening, resulting in a cost of $24,700 per quality-adjusted life-year saved. However, under conditions in which there is a relatively high prevalence of BE, high-grade dysplasia, or adenocarcinoma, low false-positive rates of endoscopy with biopsy and low reduction in quality of life with esophagectomy may not reflect the real situation and any variation of these factors make this strategy cost-ineffective. In another study, a single screening examination of subjects at 50 years of age with GERD symptoms resulted in an associated incremental cost-effectiveness ratio of $10,440 compared with no screening.[31] However, because the analysis was sensitive to the prevalence of BE and adenocarcinoma of the esophagus at the time of screening, the incidence of cancer among patients with BE and a change in parameters could make such a screening cost-ineffective. Because there are no definite data regarding how to identify subgroups of patients with BE who are more likely to develop cancer, we continue to rely on unproven mathematical models to evaluate cost-effectiveness of screening.

The purpose of screening is to detect the disease during the preclinical phase and alter its natural course before symptoms appear. Some studies indicate that subjects whose cancers are detected in screening have an improved prognosis compared with those presenting symptomatically.[32,33] Because survival in EAC is strongly correlated with stage at diagnosis,[34] finding a lesion in the early stage may confer improved prognosis. There are no randomized trials of screening programs to substantiate that endoscopic screening confers a superior life expectancy. One study was conducted to determine the prevalence of BE and possible associated risk factors in a Swedish population in which a random sample of the adult population was surveyed. The study showed that the prevalence of BE was 1.6% in a general population and 43.7% of subjects with BE had no reflux symptoms. This data suggested that a screening program based on reflux symptoms is inadequate to detect BE. For screening to be performed effectively, we need to identify asymptomatic patients with BE, so that we can detect the majority of patients with BE. This major challenge in developing an effective screening strategy for BE led to consensus that screening for BE in the general population cannot be recommended at the current time.

SURVEILLANCE

Endoscopic surveillance for patients with BE is recommended due to several crucial assumptions: the establishment of the association of BE with adenocarcinoma, the slow progression of BE through dysplasia to adenocarcinoma, the rapidly rising rate of incidence of adenocarcinoma, the dismal prognosis of adenocarcinoma when detected symptomatically, and the improved prognosis with treatment of dysplasia/neoplasia detected by surveillance. It is thought that BE sequentially progresses from no dysplasia through to low-grade dysplasia, to high-grade dysplasia and to EAC. The time-course of the progression is thought to require years and therefore a surveillance program seems to be a suitable option to detect the disease in a treatable stage. It now appears that not all BE cases progress to adenocarcinoma. Initial reports estimated the risk of developing adenocarcinoma from BE was 1% or more per year. However, several recent studies suggest that this risk was overestimated and the actual rate is approximately half that amount.[17,35–37] It is unclear whether BE decreases survival of patients compared with the patients without BE. Previous studies did not show adenocarcinoma arising from BE as having a significant impact on prognosis[38,39] and one long-term prospective observational study showed no significant overall survival between subjects with BE compared with appropriately matched individuals in the general population.[40] A major limitation of these studies was the predominant composition of elderly people who may have died of other comorbidities. Long-term studies of younger patients with BE is needed to evaluate its impact on survival and that kind of study would likely show a reduction in life expectancy. At the current time, histologic evidence of dysplasia is used as the primary means to discriminate high-risk patients.

There is still controversy on the effectiveness of surveillance endoscopy for patient-outcome. Previous studies showed that esophageal cancers detected in subjects with BE on a surveillance program were associated with longer survival than those diagnosed during evaluation of cancer symptoms.[33,41] However, the outcome of these studies may have been influenced by lead-time bias, length bias, and selection bias due to characteristics of BE and EAC.[42] Lead-time bias means that longer survival from EAC in patients undergoing surveillance endoscopy may reflect an earlier detection of incurable EAC at a very early stage without any true improvement in the overall survival. Length bias means patients with slow-growing cancers tend to have longer survival that is independent of any benefit from a surveillance program. Elderly patients or patients with significant comorbidity are less likely to be enrolled in a surveillance program and patients enrolled in such a program might have healthier lifestyles or might pay more attention to their health, which may cause selection bias. Those previous small cohort studies also suggested that only a minority of subjects with BE actually died of EAC and that the majority of people with BE died of causes other than EAC. However, a retrospective population-based cohort study of endoscopic surveillance in 23 subjects with BE among 589 subjects with adenocarcinoma showed improved survival benefit among subjects with surveillance-detected cancer.[19] Eleven of 15 subjects who were diagnosed with cancer while in a surveillance program were alive, compared with none of eight subjects who were not under surveillance. None of the deaths in the surveillance-detected patients were from cancer, compared with four deaths from cancer in the non-surveillance-detected patients. There are no prospective randomized studies that have evaluated the efficacy of surveillance in preventing EAC and its related mortality in patients with BE.

Nearly all surveillance in the United States is performed with endoscopy and biopsies.[43,44] Although there are no definite criteria as to which patients with BE should begin a surveillance program, the current recommendations are based on age, likelihood of survival over the next 5 years, the patient's understanding of the process and its limitations for detection of cancer, and the willingness of the patient to adhere to recommendations.[15] Because initial endoscopy is performed on symptomatic patients, there is a possibility of erosive esophagitis and with it the potential to reduce the detection rate by interfering with the visual recognition of BE. Therefore, patients undergoing endoscopy for detection of BE should be treated with acid-suppressive therapy before endoscopy.[45]

There is also no standardized technique for endoscopic mucosal biopsy. An assessment of the use of jumbo biopsy forceps in a surveillance program to detect unsuspected carcinoma at esophagectomy in BE patients with high-grade dysplasia showed no statistical differences in the rate of unsuspected cancers found at esophagectomy compared with standard biopsy forceps.[46] All mucosal irregularities in BE such as erosions, nodules, and strictures are sampled due to their association with an increased rate of malignancy. Based on the fact that the distribution of the dysplasia and cancer is usually patchy in BE,[47] four quadrant biopsies every 2 centimeters from the Barrett's segment, which starts at the gastroesophageal junction and stops at the squamocolumnar junction, are commonly used. Further, in the presence of high-grade dysplasia, four quadrant biopsies every centimeter are recommended to reduce the likelihood of missing coexisting cancers.[47,48] Surveillance intervals are recommended based on grades of dysplasia (Table 1). One study was conducted to assess whether endoscopic mucosal resection can be used in the diagnosis of lesions within BE whose endoscopic appearance raise suspicion of carcinoma or high-grade dysplasia.[49] The study of 25 subjects showed endoscopic mucosal resection of suspicious lesions diagnosed 13 subjects (52%) with superficial EAC and four subjects (16%) with high-grade dysplasia. It is currently accepted that patients with mucosal abnormalities that raise suspicion of advanced lesions should undergo endoscopic mucosal resection to increase detection of advanced lesions. In a retrospective study of 76 subjects with high-grade dysplasia who had no evidence of cancer on an initial evaluation, the 5-year cumulative incidence of EAC among them was 59%.[50] Another retrospective study found EAC in 14% of subjects with focal high-grade dysplasia, defined as the detection of high-grade dysplasia in fewer than five mucosal crypts in a single biopsy specimen, and in 56% of subjects with diffuse high-grade dysplasia in a 3-year observational period. Subjects with focal high-grade dysplasia demonstrated longer survival than subjects with diffuse high-grade dysplasia. This study also showed that nodularity on endoscopy was associated with a 2.5-fold increased risk of EAC.[51] A noteworthy fact for evaluating an appropriate surveillance program is that even if the initial two endoscopies lack evidence of dysplasia, there is no

Table 1		
Surveillance interval[15]		
Dysplasia	**Documentation**	**Follow-Up**
None	Two EGD[a] with biopsy within 1 year	EGD every 3 years
Low-grade	Highest grade on repeat EGD with biopsies within 6 months	1 year interval until no dysplasia × 2
High-grade	Repeat EGD with biopsies to rule out EAC within 3 months	Continued 3-month surveillance or intervention based on each case

Am J Gastroenterol 2008; 103:788–97.
[a] EGD, esophagogastroduodenoscopy.

guarantee that the patient will not develop EAC. One multicenter cohort study showed more than half of the subjects who developed EAC had no dysplasia on their first endoscopies.[52] This phenomenon might partially be explained by the limitation of the biopsy protocols; however, it still has an impact on patient follow-up.

The risk of progression from low-grade dysplasia to high-grade dysplasia to EAC in patients with BE varies. One possible explanation of the reported disparities may be interobserver variability. Low-grade dysplasia has a wide range of interpretations even with an expert gastrointestinal pathologist. A patient with a consensus diagnosis of low-grade dysplasia among pathologists has a greater likelihood of neoplastic progression.[53] Pathologic assessment remains the foundation of clinical decision making in the evaluation of the risk of progression to invasive EAC in patients with BE. In one study, intraobserver and interobserver agreements were assessed by expert gastrointestinal pathologists.[54] In this study, when statistical analysis was performed using two broad diagnostic categories (Barrett's mucosa without dysplasia/indefinite for dysplasia/low-grade dysplasia versus high-grade dysplasia/carcinoma), intraobserver agreement was good (mean $k = 0.82$ and 0.80) and interobserver agreement was moderate ($k = 0.66$ and 0.70). When the analysis was performed using four separations (Barrett's mucosa without dysplasia, indefinite for dysplasia/ low-grade dysplasia, high-grade dysplasia, and carcinoma), the intraobserver was moderate ($k = 0.64–0.68$) and the interobserver was fair ($k = 0.43–0.46$) with reasonable agreement. This study showed improved reproducibility after holding a consensus diagnostic meeting among pathologists; however, the study made it clear that distinction between low-grade dysplasia and high-grade dysplasia and between high-grade dysplasia and carcinoma was still difficult.

The cost-effectiveness of surveillance has been analyzed in several studies using mathematical models. In one study, a computer cohort of 55-year-old subjects with BE without any evidence of dysplasia were evaluated using surveillance strategies that ranged from no surveillance to surveillance every 1–5 years.[55] With an average annual incidence of cancer of 0.4%, surveillance every 5 years was found to be more cost-effective than every 1-4 years, and the incremental cost/utility ratio for surveillance every 5 years was 98,000 quality-adjusted life-years gained, comparable with incremental cost-effectiveness ratios of accepted practices. Another study assessed the cost-effectiveness of surveillance endoscopy every 2 years using mathematical models.[56] The incremental cost-effectiveness of biannual endoscopy was $16,695 per life-year saved compared with no surveillance. A more recent study assessed the cost-effectiveness of surveillance only to BE patients with dysplasia at the initial examination.[31] The strategy yielded an incremental cost-effectiveness ratio of $10,440 compared with no screening or surveillance. Although these economic analyses were well constructed and implied the cost-effectiveness of surveillance, they were sensitive to the prevalence of BE and EAC during surveillance, the incidence of cancer among patients with BE, and the mortality and health-related quality of life of surgical therapy for BE-associated cancer.

Several other methods have been studied to perform surveillance because there are latent problems associated with the use of biopsies as tools for monitoring patients with BE, including limited sampling of the affected mucosa, poor ability of histologic findings to predict which patients are likely to progress to EAC, and interobserver reproducibility among pathologists for diagnosis of dysplasia. Brush cytology has been assessed as a complementary method to standard biopsy in a couple of studies.[57,58] Advantages of cytology include its simplicity and relatively low cost, and the ability to sample a greater area of involved mucosa and cytology may reveal abnormalities missed by standard biopsy. In an early study, 65 concurrent biopsy and cytology specimens were analyzed in subjects with BE and there was a 72% (47/65) concordance between the two diagnostic techniques.[58] In 13 of the 18 discrepancies, the cytologic diagnosis had a higher diagnostic category than the concurrent biopsy and two adenocarcinomas were diagnosed cytologically in the cases in which biopsy specimens were negative for dysplasia and adenocarcinoma. Despite these possible advantages, cytology is used by only limited numbers of gastroenterologists and, until now, limited data were available on the usefulness of cytology in the surveillance of BE. One potential way to improve the efficacy of cytology is to add an objective assessment tool such as biomarkers to routine cytologic specimens. Fluorescence in situ hybridization (FISH) has been increasingly used to facilitate the diagnostic accuracy of cytologic specimens, especially for the detection of bladder cancer in urine specimens. It is also used to detect malignancies in endoscopic brushing specimens of the biliary tract, and has been studied in EAC from Barrett's esophagus. The FISH technique uses fluorescently labeled DNA probes to detect chromosomal alterations in cells. Because abnormal cells generally contain chromosomal alterations, FISH should be able to detect cells that have chromosomal abnormalities consistent with dysplasia and neoplasia in cytology specimens.[59] A pilot study of 16 subjects with BE evaluated the feasibility of using FISH of endoscopic brush cytology using two types of chromosomal probes.[60] In the study, seven of eight adenocarcinoma cases were detected by at least one of two analyzed regions by FISH and none of the samples negative for dysplasia were abnormal for either of the two genomic regions studied. More recently, different sets of probes were assessed for the detection of dysplasia and adenocarcinoma in subjects with BE and the study showed a set consisting of probes to regions 8q24, 9p21, 17q11.2, and 20q13.2 had a sensitivity and specificity, respectively, of 70% and 89% for low-grade dysplasia, 84% and 93% for high-grade dysplasia, and 94% and 93% for esophageal adenocarcinoma.[61] This technique is a promising aid in the detection of dysplasia and adenocarcinoma and has the potential to predict which patients are likely to progress to advanced lesions even without visible mucosal abnormalities. More studies are needed to clarify how FISH would be used in the clinical management of patients with BE.

Recently, new diagnostic techniques have been introduced to improve endoscopic recognition of abnormal lesions within BE and different types of new imaging modalities have been attempted. Standard endoscopy uses reflection and absorption of the light-tissue interactions to construct an image. New optical imaging modalities apply this characteristic for constructing more detailed images, because light–tissue interactions are dependent on the structural components and abnormal lesions in tissue form different interactions from normal ones. Autofluorescence imaging and narrow-band imaging are typical for such a new imaging method. In a previous study, 60 BE subjects were screened with white-light endoscopy for lesions that raised suspicion of malignancy and were then examined by autofluorescence imaging.[62] In total, lesions in 21 subjects with early neoplasia were detected by either white-light endoscopy or autofluorescence imaging; in 14 subjects by white-light endoscopy (and also by autofluorescence imaging); and in seven subjects the lesions were detected only by autofluorescence imaging. There were 20 additional high-grade dysplasia/EAC lesions detected by autofluorescence imaging alone and eleven of these areas were detected in 14 subjects with lesions detected by white-light endoscopy. This uncontrolled study suggested the autofluorescence system improves the detection of early neoplasia in subjects with BE, though the method was associated with relatively high number of false-positive lesions. Subsequently, a study using autofluorescence and narrow-band imaging was conducted to try to reduce the high false-positive rate, and the false-positive rate was in fact reduced after combined use of autofluorescence imaging and narrow band imaging.[63] More recently, an endoscopic trimodality imaging system was used in a multicenter feasibility study.[29] In the study, relative to high-resolution endoscopy, autofluorescence imaging increased the detection of subjects with high-grade dysplasia/EAC from 53% to 90% and narrow-band imaging reduced the false-positive rate of autofluorescence imaging from 81% to 26%. This result confirmed the previous results in a single-center setting and showed promising aspects of the efficiency of the trimodality imaging system for surveillance. Future randomized crossover studies are needed to clarify the true additional value of this system for the detection of high-grade dysplasia/EAC in surveillance of BE. A newly developed confocal laser endomicroscopy has been introduced to analyze cellular and subcellular changes of the mucosal layer of the esophagus. A low-powered laser is focused onto a single point in a defined microscopic field of view; light emanating from that point is focused to a detector and light emanating from outside the illuminated spot is rejected. All detected signals from the illuminated spot are captured and the image of the scanned region is constructed digitally by measuring the light returning to the detector from successive points.[64] In a recent study, this technique was applied to the in vivo diagnosis of Barrett's epithelium and associated neoplasia.[65] Based on the comparison with in vivo confocal histology and ex vivo conventional histology from corresponding areas for 63 subjects with BE, BE and associated neoplasia could be predicted with a sensitivity of 98.1% and 92.9%, and a specificity of 94.1% and 98.4%, respectively. This promising data indicates that real-time diagnosis by confocal laser endomicroscopy followed by target biopsy may reduce the rates of sampling error and the number of biopsies needed compared with the current random biopsy protocol. More data are required to confirm the real value of this real-time endoscopic histopathology diagnostic technique.

PREVENTION

Although the lifetime risk of developing esophageal cancer is low, when the risks are applied to large communities, systemic approaches to prevention such as lifestyle modification and chemoprevention become an appealing way to decrease health risks.[66] Several risk factors have been identified for esophageal cancer and one study comprehensively examined their contributions to the cancer burden in the general population by estimating the population attributable risk (PAR), which is defined as the proportion of disease in population that is attributable to a given risk factor.[67] Smoking, body mass index above the lowest quartile, GERD with symptoms at least once per day (accounting for almost half the PAR associated with the presence of any GERD symptoms), and consumption of fruits and vegetables less than twice a day on average accounted for 39.7% (95% confidence interval [CI] = 25.6%–55.8%), 41.1% (95% CI = 23.8%–60.9%), 29.7% (95% CI = 19.5%–42.3%) and 15.3% (95% CI = 5.8%–34.6%) of EAC, respectively. In this population, 78.7% (95% CI = 66.5%–87.3%) of EAC cases could be attributed to one or more of these well-established risk factors, with smoking and body mass index contributing most. In terms of esophageal squamous cell carcinoma, smoking, alcohol consumption, and low consumption of fruit and vegetables accounted for 56.9% (95% CI = 36.6%–75.1 %), 72.4% (95% CI = 53.3%–85.5%) and 28.7% (95% CI = 11.1%–56.5%), with a combined PAR of 89.4% (95% CI = 79.1%–95.0%). Though low consumption of fruit and vegetables showed a smaller PAR than either smoking or alcohol consumption, a more recent population-based prospective cohort study of 297,651 person-years of follow-up with 116 esophageal squamous carcinomas[68] concluded that an increase in total fruit and vegetable consumption by 100 grams per day was associated with a decrease in the incidence of esophageal squamous cell carcinoma by 11% (95% CI = 1%–21%). The study showed that a few known risk factors accounted for a majority of esophageal cancers and the result indicated the incidence of esophageal cancer might be decreased by reducing the prevalence of these known risk factors.

Many chemoprevention agents have been proposed. Currently, the most attention is directed to the use of acid suppression using proton pump inhibitors (PPIs) and nonsteroidal anti-inflammatory drugs (NSAIDs). A concept of the use of PPIs for prevention is based on the fact that BE is a premalignant condition and gastroesophageal reflux is a significant risk for BE. One prospective, double-blinded, randomized study using high doses of a PPI evaluated the effect of acid suppression on a reduction of BE showed a small but statistically significant regression of BE with amelioration of reflux symptoms, confirmed by pH monitoring and subjective reporting of symptoms.[69] Another study showed normalization of intraesophageal acid exposure on pH monitoring led to more differentiation and less proliferation in BE biopsy specimens.[70] The data indicated the intriguing possibility that acid suppression could have regressed dysplasia; however, at the current time acid suppression alone has not been shown to prevent dysplasia.

At the cellular level, it has been shown experimentally that gastroesophageal reflux, which predisposes to BE, is associated with injury of the esophagus and activation of the arachidonic acid pathway in the esophagus mucosa.[71] It was also shown that cyclooxygenase (COX)-2 inhibitor suppressed proliferation in Barrett's esophageal cells and proliferation was restored by prostaglandin. Subsequently, an animal study suggested that administration of both selective and non-selective COX inhibitors decreased the development of EAC.[72] A variety of observational studies suggested aspirin/NSAIDs could protect against EAC by either preventing the development of BE or by decreasing the likelihood of BE progressing to adenocarcinoma. A meta-analysis of pooled studies found a protective association between aspirin/NSAIDs and esophageal cancer of both histologic types.[73] A recent prospective study of the relation of NSAIDs and the risk of EAC showed that hazard ratios for EAC (n = 37 cases) in current NSAID users was 0.32 (95% CI = 0.14–0.76) compared with never-users, and 5-year cumulative incidence of EAC was 14.3% (95% CI = 9.3–21.6) for never-users compared with 6.6% (95% CI = 3.1–13.6) for current NSAID users.[74] This evidence led to an ongoing phase III randomized clinical trial in the United Kingdom (AspECT trial: Aspirin Esomeprazole Chemoprevention Trial) that assesses whether intervention with aspirin results in decreased mortality or conversion rate from Barrett's metaplasia to adenocarcinoma or high-grade dysplasia.

SUMMARY

The incidence of esophageal cancer, especially esophageal adenocarcinoma, is increasing and its high mortality rate is a notable fact. Improving survival rates of this disease depend on earlier detection through screening and surveillance; however, appropriate stratification of patients for esophageal cancer risk is still difficult, as is determining treatment for individual patients. Recently developing diagnostic modalities may overcome current problems and may provide better outcomes of screening and surveillance for esophageal cancer. Biomarkers are another potential tool to improve accuracy in diagnosis of esophageal cancer and a few studies using FISH have shown promising data regarding risk stratifications of BE and EAC. Future studies will clarify the potential role of biomarkers in the field of screening and surveillance for esophageal cancer. It is important to remember the low rates of incidence of EAC arising from BE and that, although advanced lesions have poor prognosis, the majority of patients with BE have benign outcomes. Still, with an ever-increasing rate of EAC, effective chemoprevention methods need to be developed and the ongoing assessment of the role of chemoprevention is awaiting a large randomized study.

REFERENCES

1. Jamel A, Siegel R, Wald E, et al. Cancer statistics. CA Cancer J Clin 2008;58(2): 71–96.
2. Brown L, Devesa S, Chow WH. Incidence of adenocarcinoma of the esophagus among white Americans by sex, stage, and age. J Natl Cancer Inst 2008;100: 1184–7.
3. Lambert R, Hainaut P. Esophageal cancer: cases and causes (part I). Endoscopy 2007;39:550–5.
4. Shimizu M, Ban S, Odze R. Squamous dysplasia and other precursor lesions related to esophageal squamous cell carcinoma. Gastroenterol Clin North Am 2007;36:797–811.
5. Chang-Claude J, Becher H, Brettner M, et al. Familial aggregation of oesophageal cancer in a high incidence area in China. Int J Epidemiol 1997;26:1159–65.
6. Iwaya T, Maesawa C, Ogasawara S, et al. Tylosis esophageal cancer locus on chromosome 17q25.1 is commonly deleted in sporadic human esophageal cancer. Gastroenterology 1998;114:1206–10.
7. Enzinger P, Mayer R. Esophageal cancer. N Engl J Med 2003;349:2241–52.
8. Lagergren J, Bergstrom R, Lindgren A, et al. Symptomatic gastroesophageal reflux as a risk factor for esophageal adenocarcinoma. N Engl J Med 1999;340:825–31.
9. Shaheen N, Ransohoff D. Gastroesophageal reflux, Barrett's esophagus and esophageal cancer, scientific review. JAMA 2002;287:1972–81.
10. Spechler S. Barrett's esophagus. N Engl J Med 2002;346:836–42.
11. Mashimo H, Wagh M, Goyal R. Surveillance and screening for Barrett's esophagus and adenocarcinoma. J Clin Gastroenterol 2005;39:S33–41.
12. Conio M, Cameron AJ, Romero Y, et al. Secular trends in the epidemiology and outcome of Barrett's oesophagus in Olmsted County, Minnesota. Gut 2001;48:304–9.
13. Wang K, Wongkeesong M, Buttar N. American Gastroenterological Association technical review on the role of the gastroenterologists in the management of esophageal carcinoma. Gastroenterology 2005;128:1471–505.
14. Ina H, Shibuya H, Ohashi I, et al. The frequency of an early esophageal cancer in male patients with oral and oropharyngeal cancer. Cancer 1994;73:2038–41.
15. Wang K, Sampliner R. Updated guidelines 2008 for the diagnosis, surveillance and therapy of Barrett's esophagus. Am J Gastroenterol 2008;103:788–97.
16. Eisen G, Sandler R, Murray S, et al. The relationship between gastroesophageal reflux disease and its complications with Barrett's esophagus. Am J Gastroenterol 1997;92:27–31.
17. O'Connor J, Falk G, Richter J. The incidence of adenocarcinoma and dysplasia in Barrett's esophagus: report on the Cleveland Clinic Barrett's Esophagus Registry. Am J Gastroenterol 1999;94:2037–42.
18. Avidan B, Sonnenbergh A, Schnell T, et al. Hiatal hernia and acid reflux frequency predict presence and length of Barrett's esophagus. Dig Dis Sci 2002;47:256–64.
19. Corley D, Levin T, Habel L, et al. Surveillance and survival in Barrett's adenocarcinoma: a population-based study. Gastroenterology 2002;122:633–40.
20. Dulai G, Guha S, Kahn K, et al. Preoperative prevalence of Barrett's esophagus in esophageal adenocarcinoma: a systematic review. Gastroenterology 2002;122: 26–33.

21. Eisen GM, Baron TH, Dominitz JA, et al. Complications of upper GI endoscopy. American Society for Gastrointestinal Endoscopy, Practice Committee. Gastrointest Endosc 2002;55:784–93.

22. Sorbi D, Gostout C, Henry J, et al. Unsedated small-caliber esophagogastroduodenoscopy (EGD) versus conventional EGD: a comparative study. Gastroenterology 1999;117:1301–7.

23. Catanzaro A, Faulx A, Pfau P, et al. Accuracy of a narrow-diameter battery-powered endoscopy in sedated and unsedated patients. Gastrointest Endosc 2002; 55:484–7.

24. Saeian K, Staff D, Vasilopoulos S, et al. Unsedated transnasal endoscopy accurately detects Barrett's metaplasia and dysplasia. Gastrointest Endosc 2002;56: 472–8.

25. Eliakim R, Yassin K, Shlomi I, et al. A novel diagnostic tool for detecting oesophageal pathology: the PillCam oesophageal video capsule. Aliment Pharmacol Ther 2004;20:1083–9.

26. Lin O, Schembre D, Mergener K, et al. Blinded comparison of esophageal capsule endoscopy versus conventional endoscopy for a diagnosis of Barrett's esophagus in patients with chronic gastroesophageal reflux. Gastrointest Endosc 2007;65:577–83.

27. Eloubeidi M, Provenzale D. Does this patient have Barrett's esophagus? The utility of predicting Barrett's esophagus at the index endoscopy. Am J Gastroenterol 1999;94:937–43.

28. Goda K, Tajiri H, Ikegami M, et al. Usefulness of magnifying endoscopy with narrow band imaging for the detection of specialized intestinal metaplasia in columnar-lined esophagus and Barrett's adenocarcinoma. Gastrointest Endosc 2007;65:36–46.

29. Curvers WL, Singh R, Wong Kee Song LM, et al. Endoscopic tri-modal imaging for detection of early neoplasia in Barrett's oesophagus; a multi-centre feasibility study using high-resolution endoscopy, autofluorescence imaging and narrow band imaging incorporated in one endoscopy system. Gut 2008;57:167–72.

30. Soni A, Sampliner R, Sonnenberg A. Screening for high-grade dysplasia in gastroesophageal reflux disease: is it cost-effective? Am J Gastroenterol 2000; 95:2086–93.

31. Inadomi J, Samplienr R, Lagergren J, et al. Screening and surveillance for Barrett's esophagus in high-risk groups: a cost-utility analysis. Ann Intern Med 2003;138:176–86.

32. Streitz JM, Andrews CW, Ellis FH. Endoscopic surveillance of Barrett's esophagus. Does it help? J Thorac Cardiovasc Surg 1993;105:383–8.

33. Peters JH, Clark GWB, Ireland AP, et al. Outcome of adenocarcinoma arising in Barrett's esophagus in endoscopically surveyed and nonsurveyed patients. J Thorac Cardiovasc Surg 1994;108:813–22.

34. Menke-Pluymers M, Schoute N, Mulder A, et al. Outcome of surgical treatment of adenocarcinoma in Barrett's esophagus. Gut 1992;33:1454–8.

35. Conio M, Blanchi S, Lapertosa G, et al. Long-term endoscopic surveillance of patients with Barrett's esophagus. Incidence of dysplasia and adenocarcinoma: a prospective study. Am J Gastroenterol 2003;98:1931–9.

36. Shaheen N, Crosby M, Bozymski E, et al. Is there publication bias in the reporting of cancer risk in Barrett's esophagus? Gastroenterology 2000;119:333–8.

37. Drewitz D, Sampliner R, Garewal H. The incidence of adenocarcinoma and dysplasia in Barrett's esophagus: a prospective study of 170 patients followed 4.8 years. Am J Gastroenterol 1997;92:212–5.

38. Van der Veen A, Dees J, Blankenstein J, et al. Adenocarcinoma in Barrett's oesophagus: an overrated risk. Gut 1989;30:857–9.
39. Van der Burgh A, Dees J, Hope W, et al. Oesophageal cancer is an uncommon cause of death in patients with Barrett's oesophagus. Gut 1996;39:5–8.
40. Eckardt V, Kanzler G, Bernhard G. Life expectancy and cancer risk in patients with Barrett's esophagus: a prospective controlled investigation. Am J Med 2001;111:33–7.
41. Macdonald C, Wicks A, Playford R. Final result from 10-year cohort of patients undergoing surveillance for Barrett's oesophagus: observational study. BMJ 2000;321:1252–5.
42. Shaheen N, Provenzale D, Sandler R. Upper endoscopy as a screening and surveillance tool in esophageal adenocarcinoma: a review of the evidence. Am J Gastroenterol 2002;97:1319–27.
43. Gross G, Canto M, Hixson J, et al. Management of Barrett's esophagus: a national study of practice patterns and their cost implications. Am J Gastroenterol 1999; 94:3440–7.
44. Falk G, Ours T, Richter J. Practice patterns for surveillance of Barrett's esophagus in the United States. Gastrointest Endosc 2000;52:197–203.
45. Hanna S, Rastogi A, Weston A, et al. Detection of Barrett's esophagus after endoscopic healing for erosive esophagitis. Am J Gastroenterol 2006;101:1416–20.
46. Falk G, Rice T, Goldblum J, et al. Jumbo biopsy forceps protocol still misses unsuspected cancer in Barrett's esophagus with high-grade dysplasia. Gastrointest Endosc 1999;49:170–6.
47. Cameron A, Carpenter H. Barrett's esophagus, high grade dysplasia, and early adenocarcinoma: a pathological study. Am J Gastroenterol 1997;92:586–91.
48. Reid B, Blount P, Feng Z, et al. Optimizing endoscopic biopsy detection of early cancers in Barrett's high-grade dysplasia. Am J Gastroenterol 2000;95:3089–96.
49. Nijhawan P, Wang K. Endoscopic mucosal resection for lesions with endoscopic features suggestive of malignancy and high-grade dysplasia within Barrett's esophagus. Gastrointest Endosc 2000;52:328–32.
50. Reid B, Levine D, Longton G, et al. Predictors of progression to cancer in Barrett's esophagus: baseline histology and flow cytometry identify low- and high-risk patient subsets. Am J Gastroenterol 2000;95:1669–76.
51. Buttar N, Wang K, Sebo T, et al. Extent of high-grade dysplasia in Barrett's esophagus correlated with risk of adenocarcinoma. Gastroenterology 2001;120: 1630–9.
52. Sharma P, Falk G, Weston A, et al. Dysplasia and cancer in a large multicenter cohort of patients with Barrett's esophagus. Clin Gastroenterol Hepatol 2006;4: 566–72.
53. Skacel M, Petras R, Gramlich T, et al. The diagnosis of low-grade dysplasia in Barrett's esophagus and its implications for disease progression. Am J Gastroenterol 2000;95:3383–7.
54. Montgomery E, Bronner M, Goldblum J, et al. Reproducibility of the diagnosis of dysplasia in Barrett's esophagus: a reaffirmation. Hum Pathol 2001;32:368–78.
55. Provenzale D, Schmitt C, Wong J. Barrett's esophagus: a new look at surveillance based on emerging estimates of cancer risk. Am J Gastroenterol 1999;94:2043–53.
56. Sonnenberg A, Soni A, Sampliner R. Medical decision analysis of endoscopic surveillance of Barrett's oesophagus to prevent oesophageal adenocarcinoma. Aliment Pharmacol Ther 2002;16:41–50.
57. Robey S, Hamilton S, Gupta P, et al. Diagnostic value of cytopathology in Barrett's esophagus and associated carcinoma. Am J Clin Pathol 1988;89:493–8.

58. Geisinger K, Teot L, Richter J. A comparative cytopathologic and histological study of atypia, dysplasia, and adenocarcinoma in Barrett's esophagus. Cancer 1992;69:8–16.

59. Halling K, Kipp B. Fluorescence in situ hybridization in diagnostic cytology. Hum Pathol 2007;38:1137–44.

60. Falk G, Skacel M, Gramlich T, et al. Fluorescence in situ hybridization of cytologic specimen from Barrett's esophagus: a pilot feasibility study. Gastrointest Endosc 2004;60:280–4.

61. Brankley S, Wang K, Harwood A, et al. The development of a fluorescence in situ hybridization assay for the detection of dysplasia and adenocarcinoma in Barrett's esophagus. Journal of Molecular Diagnostics 2006;8:260–7.

62. Kara M, Peters F, ten Kate F, et al. Endoscopic video autofluorescence imaging may improve the detection of early neoplasia in patients with Barrett's esophagus. Gastrointest Endosc 2005;61:679–85.

63. Kara M, Peters F, Fockens P, et al. Endoscopic video-autofluorescence imaging followed by narrow band imaging for detecting early neoplasia in Barrett's esophagus. Gastrointest Endosc 2006;64:176–85.

64. Hoffman A, Goetz M, Vieth M, et al. Confocal laser endomicroscopy: technical status and current indications. Endoscopy 2006;38:1275–83.

65. Kiesslich R, Grossner L, Goetz M, et al. In vivo histology of Barrett's esophagus and associated neoplasia by confocal laser endomicroscopy. Clin Gastroenterol Hepatol 2006;4:979–87.

66. Jankowski J, Hawk E. A methodological analysis of chemoprevention in the gastrointestinal tract. Nat Clin Pract Gastroenterol Hepatol 2006;3:101–11.

67. Engel L, Chow WH, Vaughan T, et al. Population attributable risks of esophageal and gastric cancers. J Natl Cancer Inst 2003;95:1404–13.

68. Yamaji T, Inoue M, Sasazuki S, et al. Fruit and vegetable consumption and squamous cell carcinoma of the esophagus in Japan: the JPHC study. Int J Cancer 2008;123:1935–40.

69. Peters F, Ganesh S, Kuipers E, et al. Endoscopic regression of Barrett's oesophagus during omeprazole treatment; a randomised double blind study. Gut 1999;45:489–94.

70. Ouatu-Lascar R, Fitzgerald R, Triadafilopoulos G. Differentiation and proliferation in Barrett's esophagus and the effects of acid suppression. Gastroenterology 1999;117:327–35.

71. Buttar N, Wang K, Anderson M, et al. The effect of selective cyclooxygenase-2 inhibition in Barrett's esophagus epithelium: an in vitro study. J Natl Cancer Inst 2002;94:422–9.

72. Buttar N, Wang K, Leontovich O, et al. Chemoprevention of esophageal adenocarcinoma by COX-2 inhibitions in animal model of Barrett's esophagus. Gastroenterology 2002;122:1101–12.

73. Corley D, Kerlikowske K, Verma R, et al. Protective association of aspirin/NSAIDs and esophageal cancer: a systematic review and meta-analysis. Gastroenterology 2003;124:47–56.

74. Vaughan T, Dong L, Blount P, et al. Non-steroidal anti-inflammatory drugs and risk of neoplastic progression in Barrett's oesophagus: a prospective study. Lancet Oncol 2005;6:945–52.

Genetic Variations in Esophageal Cancer Risk and Prognosis

Winson Y. Cheung, MD[a,b], Geoffrey Liu, MD, MSc[a,c,d],*

KEYWORDS

- Genetic polymorphism • Esophageal cancer • Risk
- Outcome • Prognosis

Genetic polymorphisms, which are inherited DNA sequence variations observed among different individuals in a population, are common enough to affect at least 1% of a specific population.[1–3] Single nucleotide polymorphisms (SNPs) are the simplest and one of the most common polymorphisms, accounting for a large proportion of the possible genetic code variations that occur within the human genome.[4,5] SNPs may fall within coding sequences of genes, noncoding regions of genes, or in the intergenic areas between genes. Of the SNPs that occur within a coding sequence, only a portion of these polymorphisms ultimately contribute to changes in the amino acid sequence of the protein that is being produced. Such SNPs are known as nonsynonymous SNPs and may culminate in phenotypic changes.[6,7] Conversely, those that do not result in amino acid alterations are synonymous SNPs.[8] Among the SNPs located in noncoding regions of genes (eg, splice sites, promoter regions, or transcriptional binding sites), which are not always actively transcribed, some may still exert a phenotypic effect on the host through either indirect interactions with other genes or regulation of downstream proteins.[8]

Research related to this article was supported by grants from the Alan B. Brown Chair in Molecular Genomics at Princess Margaret Hospital, University of Toronto; the Posluns Family Foundation; the National Institutes of Health (Research Project Grant [RO1] CA 109,193); and the Canadian Institutes of Health Research. Other financial support included a Connaught award and a scholarship from the Canadian Association of Medical Oncology.

[a] Medical Oncology and Hematology, Medicine, Princess Margaret Hospital/Ontario Cancer Institute, University of Toronto, 610 University Avenue, 7-124, Toronto, ON M5G 2M9, Canada
[b] Epidemiology, Harvard School of Public Health, Boston, MA, USA
[c] Applied Molecular Oncology, Medical Biophysics, Princess Margaret Hospital/Ontario Cancer Institute, University of Toronto, 610 University Avenue, 7-124, Toronto, ON M5G 2M9, Canada
[d] Environmental and Occupational Medicine and Epidemiology, Harvard School of Public Health, Boston, MA, USA
* Corresponding author. Medical Oncology and Hematology, Medicine, Princess Margaret Hospital/Ontario Cancer Institute, University of Toronto, 610 University Avenue, 7-124, Toronto, ON M5G 2M9, Canada.
E-mail address: geoffrey.liu@uhn.on.ca (G. Liu).

Gastroenterol Clin N Am 38 (2009) 75–91
doi:10.1016/j.gtc.2009.01.009
0889-8553/09/$ – see front matter

SNPs appear to influence the risks and outcomes of certain diseases. In some instances, SNPs predict the degree of response to particular therapeutic interventions. SNP research has been especially prominent in the field of oncology for two main reasons. The first is because prognosis for many cancers remains poor. It is thus hoped that SNP research will lead to better outcomes. SNP research has also received attention in the field of oncology because the therapeutic index of treatments is often narrow and the risks of life-threatening toxicities can be substantial, making the ability to predict risks and outcomes of cancers particularly appealing. Because of the potential predictive and prognostic power that SNPs may offer, many molecular biologists and epidemiologists hope that SNPs will soon make "personalized medicine" possible, enabling interventions to be tailored to specific patient populations. Thus far, most current research has been devoted to comparing SNPs of matched cohorts with the disease of interest to the SNPs of matched cohorts without the disease of interest. These risk analyses have shown promising but inconclusive results. Meanwhile, researchers face the challenge of deciding just which SNPs are relevant enough to study. Only a small proportion of the more than 3 million SNPs in the human genome have demonstrated actual clinical relevance. Even so, there are still many from which to choose.

The presence of other forms of genetic variations, including microsatellite instability and chromosomal insertions, deletions, and duplications, adds another layer of complexity to our understanding of SNPs. Microsatellites are short repetitive DNA sequences that are scattered throughout the genome; variations in the frequency of sequence repetitions cases instability in these sequences—microsatellite instability—is associated with many sporadic and familial cancers.[9–11] For example, CACA-CACACA or $(CA)_5$ is a conventional dinucleotide repeat in a normal cell. By comparison, in the case of an intron 1 *EGFR* polymorphism, individuals can have between 14 and 23 repeats (ie, $[CA]_{14}$ to $[CA]_{23}$). These unusual patterns correlate with cancer risk.[12] In addition, there exist chromosomal insertions and deletions that can be as small as only a few base pairs in length, but can also be as large as an entire gene, as is the case with glutathione S-transferases (eg, *GSTM1* and *GSTT1* deletions).[13] Copy number variation refers to duplication (often by many fold) or deletion of a large segment of DNA (>1 kilobases) that can encompass one or more genes. Like SNPs, each of these different germline genetic variations can affect the risk of developing cancer and the prognosis following cancer diagnosis.

The genetic factors that contribute to the pathogenesis of cancer can be either tumor-specific (eg, somatic *p53* mutation) or inherited (eg, germline *p53* mutation in Li-Fraumeni syndrome).[14,15] This review focuses on the germline/inherited variations. Inherited genetic factors, in conjunction with their interactions with other clinical variables, can alter the efficacy of the various intracellular pathways that ultimately result in carcinogenesis. For esophageal squamous cell carcinomas (ESCCs), important clinical risk factors include alcohol and tobacco exposure and local physical trauma. Meanwhile, for esophageal adenocarcinomas (EACs), clinical risk factors consist of gastroesophageal reflux disease (GERD), Barrett's esophagus, and obesity.[16,17] The interplay between genes and these clinical variables are referred to as gene–environment interactions.[18,19] Genes and the factors affecting genes represent the foundation of the emerging field of molecular epidemiologic research.

Genetic polymorphisms may act as molecular markers that can provide important predictive and prognostic information about cancers. In fact, numerous polymorphisms in several oncological settings have already been identified, including those involving breast, lung, colon, and ovarian cancers.[20–24] In this review article, we specifically focus on the clinical and research implications that genetic polymorphisms may pose for esophageal cancers. In particular, we discuss the current state of the literature with regards to genetic polymorphisms and their association with esophageal cancer risk and prognosis, and also highlight some of the potential future directions in this novel field.

POLYMORPHISMS AND ESOPHAGEAL CANCER RISK

Currently, ESCC and EAC represent the predominant tumor types that comprise the majority of esophageal cancer cases. Interestingly, while the incidence of ESCC is declining, the incidence of EAC continues to increase steadily. EAC is now the most common malignant histology affecting the esophagus.[25] In North America, the annual rate of EAC has increased dramatically three- to four-fold in the last 3 decades alone.[26,27] The prognosis of EAC remains poor, however, with 5-year overall survival rates approximating 10% to 15% only despite the use of local endoscopic treatments, new surgical techniques, and aggressive multimodality approaches that incorporate chemotherapy and radiation.[28]

In addition to the many established clinical risk factors for esophageal cancers, such as alcohol, smoking, and GERD, familial aggregations of esophageal cancers have frequently been described.[29,30] Similar familial clustering of Barrett's esophagus, a known determinant of esophageal cancer, has also been observed.[31] Likewise, those with a family history of esophageal cancer have an increased risk of the disease.[32] Whether these patterns simply reflect common environmental exposures among family members or actual inherited predispositions is uncertain, but the patterns suggest that genetic factors likely contribute in part to esophageal tumorigenesis. Moreover, alterations in certain key genes that govern DNA maintenance and repair have already been linked to elevated risks of developing various cancers, including malignancies of the esophagus.[33–36] The real uncertainty, however, lies in the precise interrelationship between genetic and environmental variables, which is purportedly more complex because only a small proportion of people with either genetic or environmental factors ultimately develop EAC. This observation suggests that there are most likely additional parameters and interactions that are crucial to esophageal carcinogenesis.

There is mounting interest in clarifying the role that genetic factors play in cancer susceptibility. Much of this interest has arisen because of recent advances and more widespread availability of high-volume, low-cost genetic analysis programs as well as easier accessibility to detailed genomic information from the Human Genome Project and other related databases.[37,38] It is hoped that better understanding of the molecular epidemiologic mechanisms that underlie the risk of developing esophageal cancer will enable clinicians to identify the most susceptible patients. In turn, this group of individuals would be expected to derive the most clinical benefit from strategies aimed at risk reduction, screening, and chemoprevention. An understanding of the genetic basis of esophageal cancer will ultimately facilitate the development of novel therapeutic approaches.

Most molecular epidemiologic research to date has focused on large-scale genome-wide studies exploring the simple association between genes and disease. These studies have been instrumental in the elucidation of specific alleles and gene loci that confer elevated risks for a diverse array of medical conditions. Most of these studies have been developed and performed under the auspices of international consortia or large collaborative groups that permit the inclusion of a large and representative patient population. This design allows for greater statistical power and, consequently, makes generalizations of the results more valid. Unfortunately, studies of genetic risk factors specific to the esophageal cancer setting have been noticeably more limited. Published literature in this area has been primarily confined to small, case-control studies. While some of these preliminary investigations have been quite successful in identifying genetic polymorphisms that warrant further study and in provoking hypotheses-generating findings, only a few putative genes have been analyzed to date. A recent systematic review indicated that fewer than 100 publications and only three small meta-analyses available in the published literature describe the genetic polymorphisms and their associations with esophageal cancer risk.[36] Esophageal cancer is also unique in that the two main histologic subtypes, ESCC and EAC, are quite distinct in most respects, including their epidemiology, clinical features, and pathogenesis. Therefore, prior papers have typically chosen to analyze these histologies separately with the majority devoted preferentially to the study of ESCC.

Esophageal Squamous Cell Carcinoma Risk

Considering that the incidence of ESCC is particularly high in parts of China and Japan, the majority of molecular epidemiologic studies have understandably taken place in the Asian population. Our previous knowledge of the environmental risk factors for ESCC, including smoking, alcohol, nitrosamine exposure, micronutrient-deficient diets, and human papillomavirus infection, has helped to shape many of these molecular epidemiologic studies.[39–42] For instance, studies have generally evaluated genetic polymorphisms involved in enzymatic processes or intracellular pathways that modulate the effects of these environmental exposures. **Table 1** summarizes these findings.

Enzymes of particular interest have included those that participate in either carcinogen activation or detoxification, such as phase I enzymes (eg, cytochrome P450

Table 1
Genetic polymorphisms and their association with risk of ESCC

Enzymes	Positive Association Studies	Positive & Negative Association Studies	Negative Association Studies
Phase I enzymes	CYP1A1 *1/*2[43,44,48] CYP3A5 *1/*3[47]	—	CYP2E1 c1/c2[43,46]
Phase II enzymes	NQO1 T609C[51,57,93] GSTM3 A/B[49]	SULT1A1 G213A[94]	GSTM1 A/B[43,44,48] GSTT1 Ile/Val[43,44,48] GSTP1 Ile/Val[43,44,48] mEH His113Tyr[52]
Enzymes involved in DNA repair, cell cycle, apoptosis	Fas A670 G[95] Fas-L T844C[95] MDM2 T309 G[96] ECRG1 Arg290Gln[97] ECRG1 TCA4/TCA3[98] p21 Arg31Ser[99]	p53 Arg72Pro[96,100,101] XRCC1 Arg280His[64] XPD Asp312Asn[61,62]	XRCC1 Arg194Trp[61,62] hOGG1 T911C[102] CCND1 G870A[79]
Other	ALDH2 *1/*2[46,53] ADH2 *1/*2[46,53] MTHFR C677 T[58,59] MTRR A66 G[103] COX2 G765C[104] BRCA2 G203A[101] MMP7 A181 G[65,105] MMP2 C735 T[65] SHMT1 C420 T[106] TAP2 G379A[107] LMP7 C145A[107] EGFR Arg497Lys with EGF A61 G[70]	TS 3R/2R[56,76]	MTHFR C677 T[58,59,76]

For some of the genes listed, there may have been only one positive study not yet validated in another cohort.

[CYP] family of enzymes),[43–47] phase II enzymes (eg, glutathione S-transferase [GST] family of enzymes),[44,45,48,49] nicotinamide adenine dinucleotide phosphate hydrogen (eg, quinine oxidoreductase 1 [NQO1] enzymes),[50,51] microsomal epoxide hydrolase (eg, mEH);[52] and those that participate in alcohol metabolism (eg, aldehyde dehydrogenases [ALDH2] and alcohol dehydrogenase [ADH2])[53–55] and folate metabolism (eg, thymidylate synthase [TS][56,57] and methylenetetrahydrofolate reductase [MTHFR]).[58,59] Another group of candidate genes that have generated tremendous scientific interest are those involved in cell cycle regulation, DNA repair, and apoptosis (eg, p53, cyclin D1 CCND1),[60] nucleotide excision repair (NER) genes, and base excision repair (BER) genes.[61–64] All of these genes have been shown to play a critical role in governing susceptibility to carcinogenic exposure, cellular response to these exposures, or subsequent ability for cellular repair and cell programmed cell death following DNA damage. However, none have been consistently shown to affect ESCC risk.

The matrix metalloproteinases (MMP) genes serve as good examples of a pathway that plays important roles in tumor invasion and metastasis through degrading extracellular matrix components.[65,66] Variations in the DNA sequence in MMP genes may contribute to altered MMP production or activity. Therefore, these genetic alterations may in turn modulate an individual's susceptibility to cancer, such as ESCC. Indeed, studies in the Chinese population have found significant differences in the genotype and allele distributions of the P574R polymorphism of MMP-9 among ESCC cases and controls.[65,66] For instance, the P574R GG genotypes were consistently associated with a significantly increased risk of ESCC as compared with the CC genotypes (odds ratio [OR] 4.08).[65,66]

In a similar manner, epidermal growth factor (EGF) has been implicated in cell proliferation and differentiation, and alterations or overexpression of EGF has been shown to be associated with a higher risk of thoracic and gastrointestinal malignancies.[67–69] Specifically, genetic polymorphisms in EGFR 497 Arg > Lys and EGF +61A > G have been shown to influence cell cycle progression, apoptosis, angiogenesis, and metastasis.[70] Interestingly, while the EGF +61A/A genotype has been noted to be significantly associated with risk of ESCC (OR 1.70), there is no clear association for the EGFR 497Arg/Arg genotype and ESCC risk.[70] This observation highlights the complexity of genetic polymorphisms in that only a subset of them is ultimately responsible for an effect or association even though all of the genes are involved in the particular carcinogenesis pathway.

One of the most consistent pieces of evidence in support of the significance of polymorphisms in ESCC risk involves the aldehyde dehydrogenase gene (ALDH2), which is the gene responsible for the elimination of acetaldehyde, a product of alcohol metabolism, from the body.[71,72] Individuals with the ALDH *1/*2 heterozygous genotype experience a substantial increase in ESCC risk with an estimated OR of 3.2.[73] This particular polymorphism, which is prevalent among East Asians but otherwise rare in other populations, codes for an inactive enzyme that results in elevated serum acetaldehyde levels after consumption of alcohol. Clinically, it is also associated with a flushing reaction following alcohol use. More importantly, this polymorphism provides proof of a gene–environment interaction since the increased ESCC risk observed with ALDH *1/*2 heterozygous genotype is strongly dependent on the degree of alcohol consumption.[73] Conversely, the homozygous *2/*2 variant is associated with a lower risk of ESCC, which has been attributed to the complete intolerance to alcohol that occurs among individuals with this genotype.[73]

Another example that illustrates the importance of gene–environment interactions involves the C677 T polymorphism of the gene for methylenetetrahydrofolate reductase (MTHFR).[58,74–76] The TT and TC genotypes of the MTHFR C677 T were observed to significantly increase the risk of both esophageal squamous cell dysplasia (OR 2.25) and ESCC (OR 1.58) when compared with the *CC* genotype.[74] Notably, a strong interaction was observed between the *TT* and *TC* genotypes and established risk factors for ESCC, such as alcohol drinking, smoking, and family history.[74] As a result, individuals with these genotypes in combination with the risk factors possessed an even greater risk for dysplasia and ESCC. Despite the strength of some of these results, however, few genes and interactions have been consistently shown to correlate with ESCC susceptibility across different studies. Unfortunately, such contradictory findings hinder our ability to derive any definitive conclusions from these data.

Esophageal Adenocarcinoma Risk

In contrast to ESCC, relatively little has been published on molecular epidemiologic patterns for EAC. Results from positive studies and details of the specific polymorphisms are summarized in **Table 2**. Approximately 24 genetic polymorphism associations with EAC risk have been reported to date. Consistent with the literature on the classic epidemiologic features (eg, incidence proportion, prevalence rates) for EAC, studies of molecular epidemiology have focused primarily on the North American and European patient populations. Again, the number of cases in the majority of these studies has been small, ranging from as few as 50 to approximately 300.[49,77–79] As with ESCC, the polymorphisms selected for study have usually involved DNA repair genes (eg, *XPC*, *XPD*, and *ERCC1*), cell cycle control and *p53* pathway genes (eg, cyclin D1 and *p73*), and phase I and II enzymes involved in carcinogen activation or detoxification (eg, *GSTT1*, *GSTP1*, and *GSTM3*).[49,77–80]

Vascular endothelial growth factor (VEGF) has also generated substantial interest among researchers. VEGF is a major regulator of angiogenesis in the process of tumor growth and metastasis. Polymorphisms in the VEGF gene have been associated with altered VEGF expression and plasma VEGF levels. As expected, preliminary investigations have discovered that functional polymorphisms in the VEGF gene (eg, −460C/T and +936C/T) are correlated with EAC risk.[81] Compared with the +936CC genotype, for instance, the +936CT and TT genotypes were significantly associated with increased risk of developing EAC (OR 1.49).[81] Furthermore, the −460CT +CC were associated with

Table 2
Genetic polymorphisms and risk of EAC

Gene of Interest	Single Nucleotide Polymorphism	Predominant Ethnicity of Patient Population
XPC[108]	Intron 9 poly(AT) insertion	White
XPD[80,108,109]	Lys751Gln	White
Cyclin D1[79,110]	G870A	White
P73[111]	5'UTR G4A + C14 T	White
GSTT1[44,49,112,113]	Deletion (*1 → *2)	White
GSTP1[44,49,112,113]	Ile104Val	White
GSTM3[77]	*A → *B	Indian
NQO1[51,93]	C609 T	White
ADH3[46,53]	*1 → *2	White
VEGF[81]	460C/T, +405C/G, and +936C/T	White
MGMT[33]	rs12268840 and I143 V	White
EGF[82]	A61 G	White
ERCC1[80]	C8092A and 118C/T	White

For some genes, more than one SNP was evaluated.

increased risk of EAC only in smokers (OR 1.57), while the $-460CT+TT$ were associated with decreased risk of EAC (OR 0.47) only in nonsmokers.[81] Compared with nonsmokers with the $+460TT$, smokers with the $+460CT+CC$ had significantly higher risk of EAC (OR 3.32), confirming the presence of a gene–environment interaction.[81] Similarly, studies of the EGF A61 G polymorphism indicate that the G/G genotype poses an increased EAC risk with an OR of 1.81. This risk is even higher in the subgroup of EAC patients with concurrent GERD or Barrett's esophagus (OR 2.18), again pointing to the presence of a gene–environment interaction.[82]

The DNA repair protein O(6)-methylguanine-DNA methyltransferase (MGMT) is the major cellular defense against alkylating DNA damage. Each of the five different MGMT SNPs (eg, rs12269324, rs12268840, L84F, I143 V, K178R) conferred increased risks of EAC.[33] Strong associations were found for the two variant MGMT alleles, rs12268840 and I143 V. Providing additional support for the significance of gene–environment interactions, homozygous carriers of MGMT rs12268840 who also suffered frequent acid reflux had significantly higher risks of EAC (OR 15.5).[33] There were similar interactions with smoking. Other DNA repair genes have also been implicated. The homozygous variant ERCC1 genotype has been associated with reduced risks of EAC, while the homozygous variant XRCC1 genotype has been observed to confer higher risks of EAC.

Unfortunately, much like studies of ESCC, studies of EAC have shown conflicting results. The lack of consistency among the various studies that often have examined the same genetic polymorphisms cannot be easily dismissed and has made the integration of the new genetic knowledge difficult. While some postulate that the variations in findings are due to possible differences in patient populations across studies, they may also be artifacts of the small sample sizes that invariably lead to high rates of false positivity. Conversely, a number of genetic polymorphisms have been reported to show no association with EAC susceptibility, but these may represent false-negative results, given the modest samples sizes of these studies.

POLYMORPHISMS AND ESOPHAGEAL CANCER PROGNOSIS

A technique to accurately estimate the outcomes of patients with esophageal cancer and to predict who might fare better with more aggressive therapies would be a powerful tool. Understandably, this possibility has generated tremendous interest among clinicians. Research into possible relationships between different genetic variants and survival among ESCC and EAC patients constitutes a new, emerging field of study. Current research aims to identify candidate genes that can be evaluated rigorously and then validated in multiple datasets. The ultimate hope is that these various genes can be used to develop prognostic models (eg, nomograms) that, in conjunction with clinical information from patients, can be summarized to provide patients and physicians meaningful prognostic information so better decisions can be made regarding management and supportive-care issues.

Overall survival rates for esophageal cancer continue to be in the range of 10% to 15% despite the aggressive use of local treatments, surgery, chemotherapy, radiation, or a combination of modalities.[28] In addition, patients who undergo these treatments frequently suffer tremendous morbidity and complications, including local toxicities (eg, dysphagia, esophagitis, disfigurement) and systemic side effects (eg, weight loss, depression), all of which can diminish quality of life.[83] Many people could benefit from a better understanding of genetic polymorphisms to potentially identify a priori individuals who might have the best chance at survival and therefore derive the most clinical benefit from treatment. Outcomes of particular scientific interest for molecular epidemiologic studies should include overall survival, recurrence and progression-free survival, response to treatment, and early and late toxicities stemming from chemotherapy and radiation.

The development of prognostic models based on genetic polymorphisms will be challenging. While a certain degree of overlap can be expected, it is possible for certain variants to have a positive effect on one outcome (eg, survival) but an opposite effect on another (eg, toxicity). For instance, nucleotide excision DNA repair pathway genes, which confer improved DNA repair capacity, may make cisplatin-based chemotherapy for non–small-cell lung cancer and ovarian cancer less effective.[84] At the same time, those same DNA repair pathway genes may help reduce the severity of side effects from exposure to platinum agents.[85]

The current literature related to polymorphisms and esophageal cancer prognosis is limited to a handful of studies (**Table 3**). Similar to studies of esophageal cancer risk, studies of esophageal cancer outcomes have been generally divided into groups based on histology and ethnicity, namely (1) analysis of genetic polymorphisms and EAC outcomes among whites and (2) analysis of polymorphic variants and ESCC outcomes among Asians. Not surprisingly, most studies to date are again limited by small sample

Table 3
Genetic polymorphisms and their association with outcomes from esophageal cancer

Gene of Interest	Single Nucleotide Polymorphism	Effect
TS[114]	TSER/6 base pair del 3' UTR	2 or 3 homozygous variants of TSER, 6 base pair del 3'UTR, and Ile105Val had better prognosis
GSTP1[114]	Ile105Val	
L-myc[90]	Intron 2 long/short	Short allele had poorer prognosis
MTHFR[89]	C677 T	No prognostic significance
TS[89]	TSER	No prognostic significance
MTR[89]	A2756 G	A/G and G/G more responsive to chemoradiation
IL-1β[115]	511	Not significant
IL-6[115]	174	C/C had reduced survival
TS[88]	6 base pair del 3' UTR	Deletion had nonsignificant improved prognosis
MTHFR[86]	A429CC222 T	G/A and A/A had better prognosis and combined variants had better prognosis
TS and MTR[86]	Multiple	"At-risk" allele combinations had worse prognosis
MDR1[86]	C3435 T	C/C and C/T had improved prognosis
NER genes[86]	9 SNPs	Decreasing number of "at-risk" alleles had better prognosis
XRCC1[86]	Arg399Gln	A/A and G/A had worse prognosis
GSTT1[116]	Deletion	No prognostic significance
GSTM1[116]	Deletion	No prognostic significance
GSTP1[116]	Ile105Val	Ile/Val and Val/Val had worse prognosis
TS[57]	G/C in TSER	2R/3 G (vs 3R/3R) genotype had 11-fold increase in lymph node metastasis in ESCC patients
TS[57]	6 base pair del 3'UTR	No prognostic significance
EGF[82]	A61 G	No prognostic significance

sizes in the form of case series and retrospective cohort studies. The majority of these studies selected overall survival and disease-free survival as the main outcome measures. In almost all of these cases, the choice of which polymorphism to analyze was determined by using preliminary information available from generic cancer-risk studies. In some cases, the decision was based on previous knowledge of potential intracellular pathways and targets believed to play important roles in carcinogenesis.

Polymorphic variants of interest come from a number of different pathways, including DNA repair (eg, *XRCC1*)[86] and xenobiotic metabolism (eg, *GSTT1*, *GSTM1*).[87] Much attention has focused specifically on pharmacogenetic pathways, particularly the folate pathway, because of the common use of 5-fluorouracil in the treatment of esophageal cancers (eg, genetic polymorphisms of thymidylate synthase and methylenetetrahydrofolate reductase).[88,89] In addition, there has also been interest in the glutathione S-transferase and DNA repair pathways because of the common use of cisplatin chemotherapy to treat esophageal tumors.[86,87] Unfortunately, no consistent pattern of results has emerged from the study of these pathways. A few polymorphic variants of other pathways (eg, *IL-1β*, *L-Myc*, *IL-6*) have also been evaluated, but only in very small studies.[90] Likewise, Wu and colleagues[86] reported a prognostic association with the polymorphic variant of the gene coding for the multi-drug-resistant protein *MDR1*. Again, independent validation of these results is neither published in the literature nor available for review.

FUTURE DIRECTIONS FOR RESEARCH

To best exploit the predictive and prognostic potential of SNPs, genetic factors and their association with esophageal cancer must be investigated in a rigorous manner. The successful and reliable identification of SNPs will only be possible if researchers employ cohort studies large enough to ensure adequate statistical power to detect true associations if they exist. This may necessitate multicenter collaborative efforts, suggesting the need to establish specialized molecular epidemiologic working groups with this focus in mind. Consensus guidelines for the design and reporting of such studies have been developed recently. These, it is hoped, should contribute to continued advances in this field.

Abiding by the principles for all scientific investigations, any positive findings in the field of molecular epidemiology and cancer should undergo blinded and independent validation by replicating studies in a separate cohort (and ideally in as many different cohorts as possible). Only pilot studies have been initiated in this area,[91,92] but larger-scale consortium efforts are ongoing. Efforts should also be undertaken to ensure the publication of methodologically sound negative findings to minimize any potential publication bias. A substantial amount of work remains to be accomplished to help identify and establish the relationships between new genetic polymorphisms and environmental exposures. Similarly, an emphasis needs to be placed on exploring potential gene–gene interactions among the different alleles that confer increased esophageal cancer risks. For example: Do SNPs that cause ESCC interact with those that cause EAC? Another promising venture is the use of DNA microarrays and "SNP chips" that can theoretically allow researchers to assess multiple genetic polymorphisms simultaneously.[91,92] This powerful technology, which can evaluate several hundred to even a million SNPs at high efficiency, enables the consideration of complex gene–gene interactions. While such novel techniques are undoubtedly beneficial, proper study design and statistical considerations continue to be of utmost importance in ensuring the validity of these high-throughput methods. Consortium-based collaborations of thousands of samples will likely define the future of this field.

The impact of genetic polymorphisms on clinical practice will likely grow as our understanding of their implications and clinical utility mature. Before we can universally incorporate their use and apply them to our patients, any genetic variants that are considered risk factors for esophageal cancer based on observational or cohort studies should ideally be evaluated in a prospective fashion. Knowledge of the patient subgroups that suffer the highest risk for developing esophageal cancer will guide management, but also calls for the use of selected screening and chemoprevention strategies to diminish the risk burden for this subset of the population.

CLINICAL IMPLICATIONS FOR RESEARCH

In part because of inconsistent results, genotypic information is not currently incorporated into common diagnostic and management algorithms for esophageal cancer, despite the increasing number of studies. While some studies have provided strongly positive findings, most were small and not performed prospectively. To ensure proper translation from clinical science to clinical practice, future studies need improved design methodology, statistical analyses, and reporting. Studies exploring the association between polymorphisms and outcomes frequently suffer from a lack of thorough reporting and often fail to include important information, such as adequate description of the source population, details of inclusion and exclusion criteria, and clinical data regarding subjects lost to follow-up and other important prognostic factors. Sound multivariate analyses are also necessary as they provide more information about the role of polymorphic variants within the larger clinical context while accounting for potential gene–gene and gene–environment interactions.

SUMMARY

The medical literature describing the role of genetic polymorphisms and their associations with risks and outcomes of cancers, including tumors of the esophagus, constitute a novel area of biomedical research. While the number of articles in this area is growing, many of the current papers suffer from methodological flaws, such as small sample sizes that lack sufficient statistical power. A movement is needed to establishment large scientific working groups that would allow for more patient enrollment in these studies. Through such collaborative approaches, the results of individual studies can be more quickly and more scientifically validated and the reasons for variations in findings now evident can be better understood. These activities will facilitate the rapid uptake of knowledge concerning genetic polymorphisms into clinical practice, which would be ideal given the significant potential benefits of a validated predictive or prognostic model for patients and their families. Finally, the next logical step in molecular epidemiologic research should emphasize the study of potential gene–gene and gene–environment interactions that will provide additional details regarding the components integral to the pathogenesis of cancers.

ACKNOWLEDGMENTS

The author's would like to thank Peggy Suen for her help in the preparation of this article.

REFERENCES

1. Efferth T, Volm M. Pharmacogenetics for individualized cancer chemotherapy. Pharmacol Ther 2005;107:155–76.

2. Nagasubramanian R, Innocenti F, Ratain MJ. Pharmacogenetics in cancer treatment. Annu Rev Med 2003;54:437–52.
3. Lee W, Lockhart AC, Kim RB, et al. Cancer pharmacogenomics: powerful tools in cancer chemotherapy and drug development. Oncologist 2005;10:104–11.
4. Dutt A, Beroukhim R. Single nucleotide polymorphism array analysis of cancer. Curr Opin Oncol 2007;19:43–9.
5. Mao X, Young BD, Lu YJ. The application of single nucleotide polymorphism microarrays in cancer research. Curr Genomics 2007;8:219–28.
6. Chorley BN, Wang X, Campbell MR, et al. Discovery and verification of functional single nucleotide polymorphisms in regulatory genomic regions: current and developing technologies. Mutat Res 2008;659:147–57.
7. Teng S, Michonova-Alexova E, Alexov E. Approaches and resources for prediction of the effects of non-synonymous single nucleotide polymorphism on protein function and interactions. Curr Pharm Biotechnol 2008;9:123–33.
8. Sauna ZE, Kimchi-Sarfaty C, Ambudkar SV, et al. Silent polymorphisms speak: how they affect pharmacogenomics and the treatment of cancer. Cancer Res 2007;67:9609–12.
9. Soussi T, Wiman KG. Shaping genetic alterations in human cancer: the p53 mutation paradigm. Cancer Cell 2007;12:303–12.
10. Zhang W, Yu YY. Polymorphisms of short tandem repeat of genes and breast cancer susceptibility. Eur J Surg Oncol 2007;33:529–34.
11. Velasco A, Pallares J, Santacana M, et al. Loss of heterozygosity in endometrial carcinoma. Int J Gynecol Pathol 2008;27:305–17.
12. Jami MS, Hemati S, Salehi Z, et al. Association between the length of a CA dinucleotide repeat in the EGFR and risk of breast cancer. Cancer Invest 2008;26:434–7.
13. Pande M, Amos CI, Osterwisch DR, et al. Genetic variation in genes for the xenobiotic-metabolizing enzymes CYP1A1, EPHX1, GSTM1, GSTT1, and GSTP1 and susceptibility to colorectal cancer in Lynch syndrome. Cancer Epidemiol Biomarkers Prev 2008;17:2393–401.
14. Tomkova K, Tomka M, Zajac V. Contribution of p53, p63, and p73 to the developmental diseases and cancer. Neoplasma 2008;55:177–81.
15. Benard J, Douc-Rasy S, Ahomadegbe JC. TP53 family members and human cancers. Hum Mutat 2003;21:182–91.
16. Pelucchi C, Gallus S, Garavello W, et al. Alcohol and tobacco use, and cancer risk for upper aerodigestive tract and liver. Eur J Cancer Prev 2008;17:340–4.
17. Yousef F, Cardwell C, Cantwell MM, et al. The incidence of esophageal cancer and high-grade dysplasia in Barrett's esophagus: a systematic review and meta-analysis. Am J Epidemiol 2008;168:237–49.
18. Taioli E. Gene-environment interaction in tobacco-related cancers. Carcinogenesis 2008;29:1467–74.
19. Edwards TM, Myers JP. Environmental exposures and gene regulation in disease etiology. Cien Saude Colet 2008;13:269–81.
20. Onay VU, Briollais L, Knight JA, et al. SNP–SNP interactions in breast cancer susceptibility. BMC Cancer 2006;6:114.
21. Kiyohara C, Takayama K, Nakanishi Y. Association of genetic polymorphisms in the base excision repair pathway with lung cancer risk: a meta-analysis. Lung Cancer 2006;54:267–83.
22. Gusella M, Padrini R. G > C SNP of thymidylate synthase with respect to colorectal cancer. Pharmacogenomics 2007;8:985–96.

23. Naccarati A, Pardini B, Hemminki K, et al. Sporadic colorectal cancer and individual susceptibility: a review of the association studies investigating the role of DNA repair genetic polymorphisms. Mutat Res 2007;635:118–45.
24. Katoh M. Cancer genomics and genetics of FGFR2 (review). Int J Oncol 2008; 33:233–7.
25. Brown LM, Devesa SS, Chow WH. Incidence of adenocarcinoma of the esophagus among white Americans by sex, stage, and age. J Natl Cancer Inst 2008; 100:1184–7.
26. Wu X, Chen VW, Andrews PA, et al. Incidence of esophageal and gastric cancers among Hispanics, non-Hispanic whites and non-Hispanic blacks in the United States: subsite and histology differences. Cancer Causes Control 2007;18:585–93.
27. Wu X, Chen VW, Ruiz B, et al. Incidence of esophageal and gastric carcinomas among American Asians/Pacific Islanders, whites, and blacks: subsite and histology differences. Cancer 2006;106:683–92.
28. Crane SJ, Locke GR 3rd, Harmsen WS, et al. Survival trends in patients with gastric and esophageal adenocarcinomas: a population-based study. Mayo Clin Proc 2008;83:1087–94.
29. Hu N, Goldstein AM, Albert PS, et al. Evidence for a familial esophageal cancer susceptibility gene on chromosome 13. Cancer Epidemiol Biomarkers Prev 2003;12:1112–5.
30. Ji J, Hemminki K. Familial risk for esophageal cancer: an updated epidemiologic study from Sweden. Clin Gastroenterol Hepatol 2006;4:840–5.
31. Chak A, Ochs-Balcom H, Falk G, et al. Familiality in Barrett's esophagus, adenocarcinoma of the esophagus, and adenocarcinoma of the gastroesophageal junction. Cancer Epidemiol Biomarkers Prev 2006;15:1668–73.
32. Akbari MR, Malekzadeh R, Nasrollahzadeh D, et al. Familial risks of esophageal cancer among the Turkmen population of the Caspian littoral of Iran. Int J Cancer 2006;119:1047–51.
33. Doecke J, Zhao ZZ, Pandeya N, et al. Polymorphisms in MGMT and DNA repair genes and the risk of esophageal adenocarcinoma. Int J Cancer 2008;123:174–80.
34. Guo W, Zhou RM, Wan LL, et al. Polymorphisms of the DNA repair gene xeroderma pigmentosum groups A and C and risk of esophageal squamous cell carcinoma in a population of high incidence region of North China. J Cancer Res Clin Oncol 2008;134:263–70.
35. Liu G, Zhou W, Yeap BY, et al. XRCC1 and XPD polymorphisms and esophageal adenocarcinoma risk. Carcinogenesis 2007;28:1254–8.
36. Hiyama T, Yoshihara M, Tanaka S, et al. Genetic polymorphisms and esophageal cancer risk. Int J Cancer 2007;121:1643–58.
37. Grant SF, Hakonarson H. Microarray technology and applications in the arena of genome-wide association. Clin Chem 2008;54:1116–24.
38. Yu K, Wang Z, Li Q, et al. Population substructure and control selection in genome-wide association studies. PLoS ONE 2008;3:e2551.
39. Freedman ND, Abnet CC, Leitzmann MF, et al. A prospective study of tobacco, alcohol, and the risk of esophageal and gastric cancer subtypes. Am J Epidemiol 2007;165:1424–33.
40. Engel LS, Chow WH, Vaughan TL, et al. Population attributable risks of esophageal and gastric cancers. J Natl Cancer Inst 2003;95:1404–13.
41. Wu AH, Wan P, Bernstein L. A multiethnic population-based study of smoking, alcohol and body size and risk of adenocarcinomas of the stomach and esophagus (United States). Cancer Causes Control 2001;12:721–32.

42. Bahmanyar S, Ye W. Dietary patterns and risk of squamous-cell carcinoma and adenocarcinoma of the esophagus and adenocarcinoma of the gastric cardia: a population-based case-control study in Sweden. Nutr Cancer 2006;54: 171–8.

43. Morita S, Yano M, Shiozaki H, et al. CYP1A1, CYP2E1 and GSTM1 polymorphisms are not associated with susceptibility to squamous-cell carcinoma of the esophagus. Int J Cancer 1997;71:192–5.

44. Abbas A, Delvinquiere K, Lechevrel M, et al. GSTM1, GSTT1, GSTP1 and CYP1A1 genetic polymorphisms and susceptibility to esophageal cancer in a French population: different pattern of squamous cell carcinoma and adenocarcinoma. World J Gastroenterol 2004;10:3389–93.

45. Nimura Y, Yokoyama S, Fujimori M, et al. Genotyping of the CYP1A1 and GSTM1 genes in esophageal carcinoma patients with special reference to smoking. Cancer 1997;80:852–7.

46. Hori H, Kawano T, Endo M, et al. Genetic polymorphisms of tobacco- and alcohol-related metabolizing enzymes and human esophageal squamous cell carcinoma susceptibility. J Clin Gastroenterol 1997;25:568–75.

47. Dandara C, Ballo R, Parker MI. CYP3A5 genotypes and risk of oesophageal cancer in two South African populations. Cancer Lett 2005;225:275–82.

48. van Lieshout EM, Roelofs HM, Dekker S, et al. Polymorphic expression of the glutathione S-transferase P1 gene and its susceptibility to Barrett's esophagus and esophageal carcinoma. Cancer Res 1999;59:586–9.

49. Jain M, Kumar S, Rastogi N, et al. GSTT1, GSTM1 and GSTP1 genetic polymorphisms and interaction with tobacco, alcohol and occupational exposure in esophageal cancer patients from North India. Cancer Lett 2006;242:60–7.

50. Li Y, Zhang JH, Guo W, et al. [Polymorphism of NAD(P)H dehydrogenase (quinone) 1 (NQO1) C 609 T and risk of esophageal neoplasm]. Zhonghua Liu Xing Bing Xue Za Zhi 2004;25:731 [Chinese].

51. Zhang JH, Li Y, Wang R, et al. [The NAD(P)H: quinone oxidoreductase 1 C609 T polymorphism and susceptibility to esophageal cancer]. Zhonghua Yi Xue Yi Chuan Xue Za Zhi 2003;20:544–6 [Chinese].

52. Lin YC, Wu DC, Lee JM, et al. The association between microsomal epoxide hydrolase genotypes and esophageal squamous-cell-carcinoma in Taiwan: interaction between areca chewing and smoking. Cancer Lett 2006;237:281–8.

53. Yokoyama A, Muramatsu T, Omori T, et al. Alcohol and aldehyde dehydrogenase gene polymorphisms and oropharyngolaryngeal, esophageal and stomach cancers in Japanese alcoholics. Carcinogenesis 2001;22:433–9.

54. Wu CF, Wu DC, Hsu HK, et al. Relationship between genetic polymorphisms of alcohol and aldehyde dehydrogenases and esophageal squamous cell carcinoma risk in males. World J Gastroenterol 2005;11:5103–8.

55. Chen YJ, Chen C, Wu DC, et al. Interactive effects of lifetime alcohol consumption and alcohol and aldehyde dehydrogenase polymorphisms on esophageal cancer risks. Int J Cancer 2006;119:2827–31.

56. Tan W, Miao X, Wang L, et al. Significant increase in risk of gastroesophageal cancer is associated with interaction between promoter polymorphisms in thymidylate synthase and serum folate status. Carcinogenesis 2005;26:1430–5.

57. Zhang J, Cui Y, Kuang G, et al. Association of the thymidylate synthase polymorphisms with esophageal squamous cell carcinoma and gastric cardiac adenocarcinoma. Carcinogenesis 2004;25:2479–85.

58. Wang LD, Guo RF, Fan ZM, et al. Association of methylenetetrahydrofolate reductase and thymidylate synthase promoter polymorphisms with genetic

susceptibility to esophageal and cardia cancer in a Chinese high-risk population. Dis Esophagus 2005;18:177–84.

59. Song C, Xing D, Tan W, et al. Methylenetetrahydrofolate reductase polymorphisms increase risk of esophageal squamous cell carcinoma in a Chinese population. Cancer Res 2001;61:3272–5.

60. Vos M, Adams CH, Victor TC, et al. Polymorphisms and mutations found in the regions flanking exons 5 to 8 of the TP53 gene in a population at high risk for esophageal cancer in South Africa. Cancer Genet Cytogenet 2003;140:23–30.

61. Xing D, Qi J, Miao X, et al. Polymorphisms of DNA repair genes XRCC1 and XPD and their associations with risk of esophageal squamous cell carcinoma in a Chinese population. Int J Cancer 2002;100:600–5.

62. Hao B, Wang H, Zhou K, et al. Identification of genetic variants in base excision repair pathway and their associations with risk of esophageal squamous cell carcinoma. Cancer Res 2004;64:4378–84.

63. Ratnasinghe LD, Abnet C, Qiao YL, et al. Polymorphisms of XRCC1 and risk of esophageal and gastric cardia cancer. Cancer Lett 2004;216:157–64.

64. Lee JM, Lee YC, Yang SY, et al. Genetic polymorphisms of XRCC1 and risk of the esophageal cancer. Int J Cancer 2001;95:240–6.

65. Yu C, Zhou Y, Miao X, et al. Functional haplotypes in the promoter of matrix metalloproteinase-2 predict risk of the occurrence and metastasis of esophageal cancer. Cancer Res 2004;64:7622–8.

66. Wu J, Zhang L, Luo H, et al. Association of matrix metalloproteinases-9 gene polymorphisms with genetic susceptibility to esophageal squamous cell carcinoma. DNA Cell Biol 2008;27:553–7.

67. Hamai Y, Matsumura S, Matsusaki K, et al. A single nucleotide polymorphism in the 5' untranslated region of the EGF gene is associated with occurrence and malignant progression of gastric cancer. Pathobiology 2005;72:133–8.

68. Lim YJ, Kim JW, Song JY, et al. Epidermal growth factor gene polymorphism is different between schizophrenia and lung cancer patients in Korean population. Neurosci Lett 2005;374:157–60.

69. Tanabe KK, Lemoine A, Finkelstein DM, et al. Epidermal growth factor gene functional polymorphism and the risk of hepatocellular carcinoma in patients with cirrhosis. JAMA 2008;299:53–60.

70. Upadhyay R, Jain M, Kumar S, et al. Interaction of EGFR 497Arg > Lys with EGF +61A > G polymorphism: modulation of risk in esophageal cancer. Oncol Res 2008;17:167–74.

71. Lee CH, Lee JM, Wu DC, et al. Carcinogenetic impact of ADH1B and ALDH2 genes on squamous cell carcinoma risk of the esophagus with regard to the consumption of alcohol, tobacco and betel quid. Int J Cancer 2008;122:1347–56.

72. Guo YM, Wang Q, Liu YZ, et al. Genetic polymorphisms in cytochrome P4502E1, alcohol and aldehyde dehydrogenases and the risk of esophageal squamous cell carcinoma in Gansu Chinese males. World J Gastroenterol 2008;14:1444–9.

73. Lewis SJ, Smith GD. Alcohol, ALDH2, and esophageal cancer: a meta-analysis which illustrates the potentials and limitations of a Mendelian randomization approach. Cancer Epidemiol Biomarkers Prev 2005;14:1967–71.

74. Li D, Diao Y, Li H, et al. Association of the polymorphisms of MTHFR C677 T, VDR C352 T, and MPO G463A with risk for esophageal squamous cell dysplasia and carcinoma. Arch Med Res 2008;39:594–600.

75. Wang J, Sasco AJ, Fu C, et al. Aberrant DNA methylation of P16, MGMT, and hMLH1 genes in combination with MTHFR C677 T genetic polymorphism in

esophageal squamous cell carcinoma. Cancer Epidemiol Biomarkers Prev 2008;17:118–25.

76. Wang L, Miao X, Tan W, et al. Genetic polymorphisms in methylenetetrahydrofolate reductase and thymidylate synthase and risk of pancreatic cancer. Clin Gastroenterol Hepatol 2005;3:743–51.

77. Jain M, Kumar S, Lal P, et al. Role of GSTM3 polymorphism in the risk of developing esophageal cancer. Cancer Epidemiol Biomarkers Prev 2007;16:178–81.

78. Murphy SJ, Hughes AE, Patterson CC, et al. A population-based association study of SNPs of GSTP1, MnSOD, GPX2 and Barrett's esophagus and esophageal adenocarcinoma. Carcinogenesis 2007;28:1323–8.

79. Casson AG, Zheng Z, Evans SC, et al. Cyclin D1 polymorphism (G870A) and risk for esophageal adenocarcinoma. Cancer 2005;104:730–9.

80. Tse D, Zhai R, Zhou W, et al. Polymorphisms of the NER pathway genes, ERCC1 and XPD are associated with esophageal adenocarcinoma risk. Cancer Causes Control 2008;19:1077–83.

81. Zhai R, Liu G, Asomaning K, et al. Genetic polymorphisms of VEGF, interactions with cigarette smoking exposure, and esophageal adenocarcinoma risk. Carcinogenesis 2008;29:2330–4.

82. Lanuti M, Liu G, Goodwin JM, et al. A functional epidermal growth factor (EGF) polymorphism, EGF serum levels, and esophageal adenocarcinoma risk and outcome. Clin Cancer Res 2008;14:3216–22.

83. Kleinberg L, Forastiere AA. Chemoradiation in the management of esophageal cancer. J Clin Oncol 2007;25:4110–7.

84. Rosell R, Taron M, Barnadas A, et al. Nucleotide excision repair pathways involved in Cisplatin resistance in non-small-cell lung cancer. Cancer Control 2003;10:297–305.

85. Selvakumaran M, Pisarcik DA, Bao R, et al. Enhanced cisplatin cytotoxicity by disturbing the nucleotide excision repair pathway in ovarian cancer cell lines. Cancer Res 2003;63:1311–6.

86. Wu X, Gu J, Wu TT, et al. Genetic variations in radiation and chemotherapy drug action pathways predict clinical outcomes in esophageal cancer. J Clin Oncol 2006;24:3789–98.

87. Harpole DH Jr, Moore MB, Herndon JE 2nd, et al. The prognostic value of molecular marker analysis in patients treated with trimodality therapy for esophageal cancer. Clin Cancer Res 2001;7:562–9.

88. Liao Z, Liu H, Swisher SG, et al. Polymorphism at the 3'-UTR of the thymidylate synthase gene: a potential predictor for outcomes in Caucasian patients with esophageal adenocarcinoma treated with preoperative chemoradiation. Int J Radiat Oncol Biol Phys 2006;64:700–8.

89. Sarbia M, Stahl M, von Weyhern C, et al. The prognostic significance of genetic polymorphisms (methylenetetrahydrofolate reductase C677 T, methionine synthase A2756 G, thymidilate synthase tandem repeat polymorphism) in multimodally treated oesophageal squamous cell carcinoma. Br J Cancer 2006;94:203–7.

90. Shibuta K, Inoue H, Sato K, et al. L-myc restriction fragment length polymorphism in Japanese patients with esophageal cancer. Jpn J Cancer Res 2000;91:199–203.

91. Hu N, Wang C, Hu Y, et al. Genome-wide association study in esophageal cancer using GeneChip mapping 10 K array. Cancer Res 2005;65:2542–6.

92. Ng D, Hu N, Hu Y, et al. Replication of a genome-wide case-control study of esophageal squamous cell carcinoma. Int J Cancer 2008;123:1610–5.

93. Zhang J, Schulz WA, Li Y, et al. Association of NAD(P)H: quinone oxidoreductase 1 (NQO1) C609 T polymorphism with esophageal squamous cell carcinoma in a German Caucasian and a northern Chinese population. Carcinogenesis 2003;24:905–9.

94. Wu MT, Wang YT, Ho CK, et al. SULT1A1 polymorphism and esophageal cancer in males. Int J Cancer 2003;103:101–4.

95. Sun T, Miao X, Zhang X, et al. Polymorphisms of death pathway genes FAS and FASL in esophageal squamous-cell carcinoma. J Natl Cancer Inst 2004;96: 1030–6.

96. Hong Y, Miao X, Zhang X, et al. The role of P53 and MDM2 polymorphisms in the risk of esophageal squamous cell carcinoma. Cancer Res 2005;65:9582–7.

97. Li Y, Zhang X, Huang G, et al. Identification of a novel polymorphism Arg290Gln of esophageal cancer related gene 1 (ECRG1) and its related risk to esophageal squamous cell carcinoma. Carcinogenesis 2006;27:798–802.

98. Yue CM, Bi MX, Tan W, et al. Short tandem repeat polymorphism in a novel esophageal cancer-related gene (ECRG2) implicates susceptibility to esophageal cancer in Chinese population. Int J Cancer 2004;108:232–6.

99. Wu MT, Wu DC, Hsu HK, et al. Association between p21 codon 31 polymorphism and esophageal cancer risk in a Taiwanese population. Cancer Lett 2003;201: 175–80.

100. Lee JM, Lee YC, Yang SY, et al. Genetic polymorphisms of p53 and GSTP1, but not NAT2, are associated with susceptibility to squamous-cell carcinoma of the esophagus. Int J Cancer 2000;89:458–64.

101. Hu N, Li WJ, Su H, et al. Common genetic variants of TP53 and BRCA2 in esophageal cancer patients and healthy individuals from low and high risk areas of northern China. Cancer Detect Prev 2003;27:132–8.

102. Xing DY, Tan W, Song N, et al. Ser326Cys polymorphism in hOGG1 gene and risk of esophageal cancer in a Chinese population. Int J Cancer 2001;95:140–3.

103. Stolzenberg-Solomon RZ, Qiao YL, Abnet CC, et al. Esophageal and gastric cardia cancer risk and folate- and vitamin B(12)-related polymorphisms in Linxian, China. Cancer Epidemiol Biomarkers Prev 2003;12:1222–6.

104. Zhang X, Miao X, Tan W, et al. Identification of functional genetic variants in cyclooxygenase-2 and their association with risk of esophageal cancer. Gastroenterology 2005;129:565–76.

105. Zhang J, Jin X, Fang S, et al. The functional polymorphism in the matrix metalloproteinase-7 promoter increases susceptibility to esophageal squamous cell carcinoma, gastric cardiac adenocarcinoma and non-small cell lung carcinoma. Carcinogenesis 2005;26:1748–53.

106. Wang YM, Guo W, Zhang XF, et al. [Correlations between serine hydroxymethyltransferase1 C1420 T polymorphisms and susceptibilities to esophageal squamous cell carcinoma and gastric cardiac adenocarcinoma]. Ai Zheng 2006;25: 281–6 [Chinese].

107. Cao B, Tian X, Li Y, et al. LMP7/TAP2 gene polymorphisms and HPV infection in esophageal carcinoma patients from a high incidence area in China. Carcinogenesis 2005;26:1280–4.

108. Casson AG, Zheng Z, Evans SC, et al. Polymorphisms in DNA repair genes in the molecular pathogenesis of esophageal (Barrett) adenocarcinoma. Carcinogenesis 2005;26:1536–41.

109. Ye W, Kumar R, Bacova G, et al. The XPD 751Gln allele is associated with an increased risk for esophageal adenocarcinoma: a population-based case-control study in Sweden. Carcinogenesis 2006;27:1835–41.

110. Geddert H, Kiel S, Zotz RB, et al. Polymorphism of p16 INK4A and cyclin D1 in adenocarcinomas of the upper gastrointestinal tract. J Cancer Res Clin Oncol 2005;131:803–8.
111. Ryan BM, McManus R, Daly JS, et al. A common p73 polymorphism is associated with a reduced incidence of oesophageal carcinoma. Br J Cancer 2001;85: 1499–503.
112. Casson AG, Zheng Z, Chiasson D, et al. Associations between genetic polymorphisms of phase I and II metabolizing enzymes, p53 and susceptibility to esophageal adenocarcinoma. Cancer Detect Prev 2003;27:139–46.
113. Casson AG, Zheng Z, Porter GA, et al. Genetic polymorphisms of microsomal epoxide hydroxylase and glutathione S-transferases M1, T1 and P1, interactions with smoking, and risk for esophageal (Barrett) adenocarcinoma. Cancer Detect Prev 2006;30:423–31.
114. Okuno T, Tamura T, Yamamori M, et al. Favorable genetic polymorphisms predictive of clinical outcome of chemoradiotherapy for stage II/III esophageal squamous cell carcinoma in Japanese. Am J Clin Oncol 2007;30:252–7.
115. Deans DA, Wigmore SJ, Gilmour H, et al. Elevated tumour interleukin-1beta is associated with systemic inflammation: a marker of reduced survival in gastro-oesophageal cancer. Br J Cancer 2006;95:1568–75.
116. Lee JM, Wu MT, Lee YC, et al. Association of GSTP1 polymorphism and survival for esophageal cancer. Clin Cancer Res 2005;11:4749–53.

Esophageal Cancer: Ultrasonography

Alan Brijbassie, MD[a], Vanessa M. Shami, MD[b],*

KEYWORDS

- Esophageal cancer • Endoscopic ultrasound
- Esophageal cancer staging
- Esophageal stricture dysphagia

Esophageal malignancy (primarily squamous and adenocarcinoma) is a major source of morbidity and mortality, despite the recently increased attention to screening and early detection. It remains as the seventh leading cause of cancer death worldwide, with a reported incidence as high as 30 to 800 cases per 100,000 persons in particular areas of northern Iran, southern Russia, and northern China. The worldwide epidemiology differs from that in the United States, with squamous cell carcinoma responsible for approximately 95% of all esophageal cancers.[1] The European-weighted survival, calculated from the pool of all cancer registries, was 33% at 1 year and 10% at 5 years.[2] The 3-year survival rate of patients with loco-regional spread after curative resection still remains low. In the United States in 2008, the American Cancer Society estimates that there will be 16,470 new cases (12,970 men and 3,500 women) of esophageal cancer diagnosed, and 14,280 persons (11,250 men and 3,030 women) are expected to die of the disease. Adenocarcinoma, as opposed to its worldwide squamous counterpart, has the fastest growing incidence rate of all cancers in the United States, with an age-adjusted incidence of 5.8 cases per 100,000 persons.[1]

Prognosis for esophageal cancer still remains grim,[3–5] with advanced tumor stage and lymph node metastases conferring even graver outcomes.[6–13] The TNM (Tumor, Lymph node and Metastasis) staging of esophageal cancer has undergone many refinements over the course of the past few years (**Box 1** and **Table 1**). Several studies have demonstrated that the addition of preoperative neoadjuvant chemoradiotherapy may improve survival in patients with locally advanced tumor (T3, -4) disease or local lymph node metastases.[14] It is here that endoscopic ultrasonography (EUS) finds its niche in the precise staging of these tumors and the subsequent use of stage-dependent treatment protocols.

[a] Carilion Clinic, 3113-G Honeywood Lane, Roanoke, VA 24018, USA
[b] Department of Medicine, Division of Gastroenterology, University of Virginia Digestive Health Center of Excellence, Box 800708, Charlottesville, VA 22908, USA
* Corresponding author.
E-mail address: vms4e@hscmail.mcc.virginia.edu (V.M. Shami).

Gastroenterol Clin N Am 38 (2009) 93–104
doi:10.1016/j.gtc.2009.01.005
0889-8553/09/$ – see front matter. Published by Elsevier Inc.

gastro.theclinics.com

> **Box 1**
> **Definitions from the TNM Classification System for esophageal carcinoma according to the American Joint Committee on Cancer Guidelines**
>
> TX–Tumor cannot be assessed
>
> T0–No evidence of primary tumor
>
> Tis–Carcinoma in situ
>
> T1–Tumor invades submucosa or lamina propria
>
> T1a–Tumor invades lamina propria
>
> T1b–Tumor invades submucosa
>
> T2–Tumor invades muscularis propria
>
> T3–Tumor invades adventitia
>
> T4–Tumor invades adjacent structures
>
> NX–Regional lymph nodes cannot be assessed
>
> N0–No regional lymph nodes involved
>
> N1–Regional lymph nodes present
>
> MX–Distant metastasis cannot be assessed
>
> M0–No distant metastasis
>
> M1a–Metastasis in the celiac lymph nodes if the tumor is in the lower one-third of the esophagus
>
> M1a–Metastasis in the cervical lymph nodes if the tumor is in the upper one-third of the esophagus
>
> M1b–Nonregional lymph nodes or other distant metastasis
>
> *From* Catalano MF, Sivak MV Jr., Rice T, et al. Endosonographic features predictive of lymph node metastasis. Gastrointest Endosc 1994;40:442–6.

EUS STAGING

EUS employs the technology of endoscopy coupled with internally placed high-frequency ultrasound waves. An ultrasound transducer mounted on the tip of the endoscope permits accurate imaging of tumors and lesions located within and adjacent to the esophagus. In addition, EUS-guided fine-needle aspiration (EUS-FNA) may be performed in adjunct to both confirm tumor diagnosis and facilitate staging.

Table 1
TNM staging for esophageal carcinoma

	TNM		Stage
Tis	N0	M0	0
T1	N0	M0	1
T2	N0	M0	IIA
T3	N0	M0	
T1	N1	M0	IIB
T2	N1	M0	
T3	N1	M0	III
T4	Any N	M0	IV
Any T	Any N	M1	

Conventional EUS has two designs: the radial scanner and the linear scanner. The 360° radial scanner produces a 360° view perpendicular to the shaft of the endoscope and has the option of scanning at 12 MHz or 7.5 MHz. The higher frequency (12 MHz) permits better visualization of details at close range; the lower frequency (7.5 MHz) serves the purpose of better ultrasound wave penetration, thus permitting a greater evaluation field. This radial echoendoscope is useful because it gives a 360° overview, similar to a computer tomogram, allowing complete visualization of the gastrointestinal tract and its adjacent structures.

The linear array sector scanner operates at 5 MHz or 7.5 MHz and has color Doppler capability useful in the imaging of vascular structures. Ultrasound scans are made parallel to the shaft of the scope and has a limited (100°) sector of scanning area. The curved linear-array design permits direct needle aspiration (FNA). These sector scanners are preferred for use in EUS-FNA because they allow direct visualization of the needle up to 5 cm to 6 cm parallel to the shaft of the endoscope.

EUS has the unique ability to image the esophageal wall as a series of definable layers corresponding to histology (T). Additionally, this technology allows identification and FNA sampling of locoregional lymph nodes (N). Distant metastases (M), as defined by the presence of positive celiac node involvement or liver metastasis, can also be adequately visualized with this technology.

T-Staging

Identification of the normal ultrasonographic layers of the esophagus allows recognition of the degree of tumor infiltration (**Fig. 1**). The first hyperechoic layer corresponds to the mucosa, the second hypoechoic layer corresponds to the muscularis mucosa, the third hyperechoic layer corresponds to the submucosa, the fourth hypoechoic layer corresponds to the muscularis propria, and the fifth hyperechoic layer corresponds to the adventitia. The clinical classification for the depth of tumor invasion (T) is assessed as follows: invasion to the second ultrasound layer (T1a), invasion up to third ultrasound layer (T1b), invasion limited to the fourth ultrasound layer (T2) (**Fig. 2**), invasion beyond the fourth ultrasound layer (T3) (**Fig. 3**), and invasion of adjacent structures such as the aorta, azygous vein, or trachea (T4).

N-Staging

Lymph node involvement is designated by either N0 or N1, corresponding to whether the node is affected (N1) or not (N0). EUS allows visualization of left paratracheal,

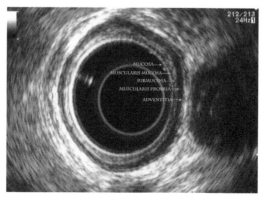

Fig. 1. Radial EUS image illustrating the normal sonographic appearance of the esophageal wall layers.

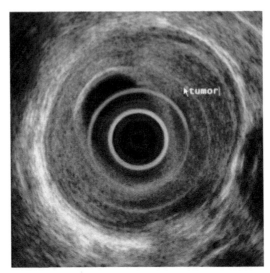

Fig. 2. Radial EUS image of an esophageal carcinoma that invades the muscle layer but does not penetrate completely through the wall (T2).

subcarinal, aortopulmonary, and paraesophageal lymph nodes. The accuracy for EUS-lymph node staging is reported to be in the range of 70% to 80%.[15] Lymph node EUS features suggestive of malignancy include size greater than or equal to 1 cm, rounded shape, well-delineated borders, and a hypoechoic internal structure (**Fig. 4**).[16,17] If all of these features are present, malignant lymph node invasion can be predicted with an accuracy of 80% to 100%. However, all four of these features are only present in one-fourth of cases, thus making it difficult to predict lymph node metastasis in the remaining three-fourths of cases. An erroneous classification

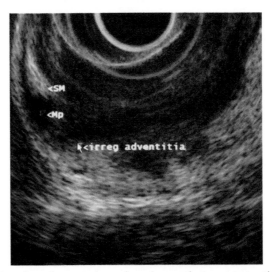

Fig. 3. Radial EUS imaging of an esophageal carcinoma that penetrates through the wall of the esophagus (stage T3).

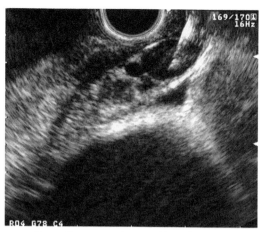

Fig. 4. Linear EUS image of a malignant peritumoral lymph node. It has all the sonographic features of malignancy including size greater than 1 cm, homogeneous, round, and with distinct borders.

for N staging has been reported at 25%, mainly because of nonspecific peritumorous inflammatory appearances.[18]

The development of EUS-FNA has increased accuracy of nodal staging.[19] In a multi-center trial of 171 patients with upper gastrointestinal lesions, EUS-FNA for N staging had a sensitivity of 92%, specificity of 92%, positive predictive value of 100%, and a negative predictive value of 96%, with an overall accuracy of 92%.[20] In another series, EUS-FNA compared with EUS had an accuracy of 87% and 74%, respectively.[21] However, there are instances where the lymph node is inaccessible without traversing the primary tumor. FNA in these cases is not recommended secondary to the risk of sample contamination and false-positive results.[22,23] The current standard of care is to perform EUS-FNA whenever feasible to maximize staging accuracy.[24,25]

M-Staging

Perhaps, the most important role EUS plays in the staging of esophageal cancer is the identification of malignant celiac lymphadenopathy. Its presence denotes M1a or stage 4 disease and usually deems patients inoperable. Celiac lymph nodes are defined by their location within a 2-cm area from the celiac trunk (**Fig. 5**). In a study by Puli and colleagues,[26] where data was extracted from 25 studies, the pooled sensitivity of EUS in the detection of celiac adenopathy was 67.2%, while the specificity was 98.1%. Reed and colleagues[27] evaluated the clinical impact of performing EUS after CT in a group of 62 patients. EUS detected abnormal celiac lymph nodes in 19 patients, with cytologic confirmation in 15. On the other hand, CT only revealed suspicious celiac lymph nodes in two patients. This enhanced detection of celiac adenopathy is crucial, as its presence portends a poor prognosis; potential unresectability, and consequently, palliation is offered. More recently, some institutions have treated M1a disease with induction chemoradiation followed by surgery with the goal of cure.[28] However, using this aggressive approach, the vast majority of these patients died secondary to their disease. Positron emission tomography (PET) has also been compared with EUS in the detection of celiac adenopathy. Flamen and colleagues[29] showed that PET significantly improved the detection of M1 disease

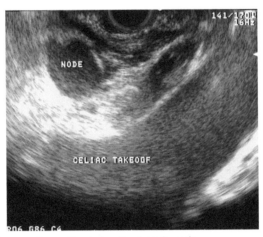

Fig. 5. Linear EUS image of a malignant celiac lymph node.

over that achieved by combination spiral CT and EUS (82% versus 64%, respectively; $P = .004$), but did not improve the accuracy of locoregional lymph-node staging (33% versus. 81%; $P = .027$).

Lastly, comprehensive EUS staging of esophageal cancer includes inspection of the liver for metastatic disease (**Fig. 6**). Studies have shown that EUS can pick up metastases, especially in the left lobe of the liver, which may not be detected by CT.[30–32] For example, the study performed by McGrath and colleagues[31] looked at 98 patients who underwent EUS staging for a new diagnosis of cardial or esophageal cancer. Of the 41 patients who underwent high-resolution helical CT scanning, EUS detected three (7%) malignant liver lesions not detected by CT. Therefore, it has been recommended that dedicated left-hepatic lobe examination should be performed in all patients undergoing upper gastrointenstinal EUS for the staging or diagnosis of malignancy. Other less frequent sites of metastases that can be detected by EUS include the left adrenal gland and malignant ascites (**Fig. 7**).

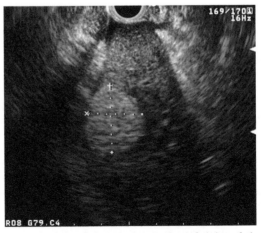

Fig. 6. Linear EUS image of a hyperechoic lesion in the left lobe of the liver representing metastasis.

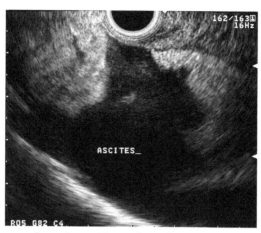

Fig. 7. Linear EUS image of a patient with esophageal cancer who has malignant ascites.

FUTURE OF EUS TECHNOLOGY

Elastography is the visualization of tissue elasticity, which can be performed during EUS. The software can be incorporated into the EUS processors. Because malignant processes tend to be harder than surrounding tissues, the elasticity is different and represented in transparent color superimposed on the EUS image.[33,34] This field is still being studied and believed to provide helpful supplementary information in identification of malignant masses and lymph nodes.

Contrast-enhanced ultrasonography is emerging as a new technique, especially in the pancreas.[35] Further data needs to be accumulated in regards to its use in other types of malignancies.

HOW GOOD IS EUS?

EUS has been compared with traditional staging modalities, such as CT, for the staging of esophageal cancer. Studies have determined that EUS is at least 50% more accurate in evaluating the T and N stages.[36,37] Numerous studies have also highlighted the unreliability of CT in differentiating stage I from stage II, or even stage III disease.[38] Thus far, EUS has been the only reliable tool in determining the extent of local disease, including spread to regional lymph nodes. Several prospective studies have demonstrated this superiority of EUS over CT scanning in T and N staging. The reported sensitivity of T staging for EUS approximates 80% to 90%, while that for N staging ranges from 70% to 80%. In contrast, the sensitivity of CT scanning has been reported to be in the range of 50% for both T and N stages. Studies have demonstrated a close correlation between EUS staging and survival rates, thereby underscoring the importance of correct preoperative staging when contemplating surgical resection.[39]

Radiologic imaging with PET or CT scanning is superior to EUS when screening for distant metastatic disease. PET scan has been stated to possibly be the most accurate tool in this setting. In one study of 100 patients with esophageal cancer, PET had a sensitivity of 69% and an accuracy of 84% in comparison to CT (45% and 63% respectively).[40] A recent prospective study of 75 patients with newly diagnosed esophageal cancer evaluated by PET, CT, and EUS found similar performance for detection of metastatic disease with PET and CT, which were both superior to

EUS.[41] PET and CT had a sensitivity of 81% and specificity of 91% and 82%, respectively, for detection of metastatic disease, compared with sensitivity of 73% and specificity of 86% with EUS. In a single-center prospective study, McDonough and colleagues,[42] revealed that PET added little information as an adjunct to EUS and CT in the initial treatment stratification of patients with esophageal cancer. From this data it can be concluded that cross-section imaging is superior to EUS in the assessment of distant metastatic disease.

EUS is not without some criticism, as this modality may involve under- as well as over-staging. Tumor micro-invasion was found to be the most important cause of tumor under-staging, whereas over-staging was mainly because of associated scar tissue that had the appearance of malignant tissue.[18] In addition, the inability of EUS to clearly distinguish between the advential and the subadvential layer is another source of error in the differentiation of T2 tumors that deeply infiltrate into the subadventia and T3 carcinomas. Further studies are required to determine whether higher ultrasound frequencies can improve the detection of tumor microinfiltration.

STAGING IN THE SETTING OF MALIGNANT STRICTURES

A technical limiting factor in EUS staging in patients with esophageal cancer is lumen obstruction. Failure to pass an echoendoscope beyond a malignant stricture is an accurate predictor of advanced T classification and poorer survival. More than 90% of patients with a nontraversable stricture have stage III or IV disease.[43] Median survival in patients with a nontraversable stricture is approximately 10 months, compared with those without a stenosis, who have a median survival of approximately 20 months.[44]

The reported incidence of stenosis precluding complete endosonographic assessment is 25% to 30%.[45,46] Dilation of the malignant stricture before EUS has been reported to result in a high-complication rate in some studies (20%).[43] However, in other studies, it appears quite safe.[47] For example, in a multicenter retrospective study with 272 cases, 28% of cases required dilation. EUS was performed with a radial echoendoscope and FNA was then performed with a curved linear echoendoscope where appropriate. Dilation was performed through at least two balloon sizes, but usually through three sizes of a single balloon without fluoroscopy. In this series, there were two perforations, one during EUS with dilation and one during EUS without dilation. The perforation associated with dilation occurred when a TTS (Through-The-Scope) balloon was inflated directly to 16.5 mm. Of patients who required dilation, 19% had celiac adenopathy, and the investigators concluded these nodes would have been missed had dilation not been undertaken. TTS balloon dilators may have advantages over bougienage because it does not require repeated esophageal intubations or fluoroscopy.

The more recent literature demonstrating the safety of EUS in stenotic tumors may in part be secondary to the slimmer and tapered newer generation instruments used in the latter study, which required less dilatation than those used in the prior Van Dam study.[43] In patients where dilation is not sufficient, there are two potential solutions for this problem:[1] the use of EUS probes that can be introduced over a guidewire and[2] the application of small radial mini-probes that can be introduced through the working channel of a conventional endoscope. Newer models of small-diameter miniprobes capable of traversing malignant strictures, while still providing good staging accuracy, are incapable of performing FNA. One potential solution to this problem would be use of the slimmer linear endobronchial ultrasound (EBUS) scope in the esophagus to FNA regional and celiac lymph nodes.

EUS RESTAGING

The accuracy of EUS for the initial staging of esophageal malignancy can hardly be questioned, but does this accuracy remain after chemoradiation therapy (CRT)? Several studies have determined that this accuracy is in fact lost, and recommendations were put forth that discouraged the technology in this setting. In a study performed by Kalha and colleagues[48] on 83 post-CRT patients, the sensitivities reported for individual T classifications were 0% for T0 tumors, 19% for T1 tumors, 27% for T2 tumors, 52% for T3 tumors, and 0% for T4 tumors. Furthermore, it was noted that when EUS results were compared with surgical pathology results, 42 patients out of the cohort were over-classified while 15 were under-classified. The results were again similar when lymph node status (N) was assessed, with EUS sensitivities for N0 and N1 disease being reported as 48% and 52%, respectively. The main reason for this considerable drop in sensitivity before and after CRT has been attributed to induction of esophageal intra-wall layer changes; changes that EUS imaging are not sensitive enough to distinguish from viable tumor. These changes take the form of inflammation and fibrosis, which lead to large artifacts on the EUS images. This discrepancy again has been highlighted in the true characterization of the difficult T2 lesions; a T2 tumor can extend to the very boundary of the muscularis propria, whereas a T3 tumor only needs to cross this boundary into the subadventitia to be classified as a non-T2 tumor.[49] This difference occurs over a very short distance, which can lead to the over-classification of T2 tumors or the under-classification of T3 tumors. This differentiation is made even worse after CRT because of the resultant peritumoral inflammation and fibrosis that serves to distort the intra-wall layers of the esophagus. Stemming from the loss of EUS sensitivity after CRT, the only viable option studied and reported by Isenberg and colleagues[50] in monitoring tumor response to therapy was the use of the actual tumor size and cross-sectional area. A response to therapy was later defined by Chak and colleagues[51] as a reduction of the cross-sectional area by 50%.

DETECTION OF TUMOR RECURRENCE

Tumor recurrence in patients who have been treated for esophageal cancer is the most common cause of mortality. Approximately 50% of patients develop recurrent disease within 2 years of surgery. Cross-sectional imaging is currently the standard for surveillance at most institutions. There are studies, however, that have shown that EUS can detect cancer recurrence with a positive predictive value of 75% to 100%.[52,53] EUS is more sensitive than endoscopy in detecting locoregional recurrence, as recurrent disease is often extra-mucosal. Additionally, EUS appears more helpful than CT in the detection of subtle lesions within or immediately adjacent to the gastrointestinal lumen. For example, in a study of 40 patients who underwent surgical resection of esophageal cancer, 10% had an unsuspected anastomotic recurrence diagnosed by EUS despite a negative CT. In another study of 43 patients undergoing routine surveillance using EUS every 6 months for at least 2 years after surgery, two-thirds did not have symptoms when recurrent disease was found. The true impact of earlier recurrent-tumor detection still needs to be elucidated because the majority of these patients have a dismal prognosis.

SUMMARY

The ability of gastroenterologists to increase survival in patients diagnosed with esophageal cancer is dependant not only upon earlier detection through adequate screening and surveillance strategies, but in precise anatomic staging that currently drives established evidence-based treatment protocols. It is in this regard that EUS finds itself the center of attention. The technology has firmly established itself as the loco-regional staging procedure of choice, and with the advent of EUS-FNA, the tide of data favors its use. The use of neoadjuvant therapy is a relatively new practice, where the selection of suitable patients is of paramount importance and it is EUS currently that sits at the cornerstone in this clinical decision-making process. Not only is it useful in identifying patients who may benefit from this therapy, but it has also been used to identify that subset of patients for whom resection/neoadjuvant therapy may not be indicated (eg, those with T4 or M1 disease). Accurate staging is crucial not only for prognosis, but for directing treatment.

REFERENCES

1. Fisichella PM, Patti MG. Esophageal cancer. Emedicine 2008, August 26th.
2. Faivre J, Forman D, Esteve J, et al. Survival of patients with esophageal and gastric cancers in Europe. Eur J Cancer 1998;34:2167–75.
3. Pera M, Cameron AJ, Trastek VF, et al. Increasing incidence of adenocarcinoma of the esophagus and esophagogastric junction. Gastroenterology 1993;104: 510–3.
4. Blot WJ, Devesa SS, Kneller RW, et al. Rising incidence of adenocarcinoma of the esophagus and gastric cardia. JAMA 1991;265:1287–9.
5. Blot WJ, McLaughlin JK. The changing epidemiology of esophageal cancer. Semin Oncol 1999;26(Suppl 15):2–8.
6. DeMeester TR. Esophageal carcinoma: current controversies. Semin Surg Oncol 1997;13:217–33.
7. Fockens P, Kisman K, Merkus MP, et al. The prognosis of esophageal carcinoma staged irresectable (T4) by endosonography. J Am Coll Surg 1998;186:17–23.
8. Korst RJ, Rusch VW, Venkatraman E, et al. Proposed revision of the staging classification for esophageal cancer. J Thorac Cardiovasc Surg 1998;115:660–70.
9. Seitz JF, Perrier H, Monges G, et al. Multivariate analysis of the prognostic and predictive factors of response to concomitant radiochemotherapy in epidermoid cancers of the esophagus. Value of immunodetection of protein p53. Gastroenterol Clin Biol 1995;19:465–74 [French].
10. Berdejo L. Transhiatal versus transthoracic esophagectomy for clinical stage I esophageal carcinoma. Hepatogastroenterology 1995;42:789–91.
11. Law SY, Fok M, Wong J. Pattern of recurrence after oesophageal resection for cancer: clinical implications. Br J Surg 1996;83:107–11.
12. Stark SP, Romberg MS, Pierce GE, et al. Transhiatal versus transthoracic esophagectomy for adenocarcinoma of the distal esophagus and cardia. Am J Surg 1996;172:478–82.
13. Pommier RF, Vetto JT, Ferris BL, et al. Relationships between operative approaches and outcomes in esophageal cancer. Am J Surg 1998;175:422–5.
14. Graham AJ, Shrive FM, Ghali WA, et al. Defining the optimal treatment of locally advanced esophageal cancer: a systematic review and decision analysis. Ann Thorac Surg 2007;83:1257–64.
15. Rosch T, Classen M. Staging esophageal cancer: the munich experience. In: van Dam J, Sivak MV Jr, editors. Gastrointestinal endosonography. Philadelphia: WB Saunders; 1999. p. 139–45.
16. Catalano MF, Sivak MV Jr, Rice T, et al. Endosonographic features predictive of lymph node metastasis. Gastrointest Endosc 1994;40:442–6.

17. Bhutani MS, Hawes RH, Hoffman BJ. A comparison of the accuracy of echo features during endoscopic ultrasound (EUS) and EUS-guided fine-needle aspiration for diagnosis of malignant lymph node invasion. Gastrointest Endosc 1997; 45:474–9.
18. Kelly S, Harris KM, Berry E, et al. A systematic review of the staging performance of endoscopic ultrasound in gastroesophageal carcinoma. Gut 2001;49:534–9.
19. Hoffman BJ, Hawes RH. Endoscopic ultrasonography-guided puncture of the lymph nodes: first experience and clinical consequences. Gastrointest Endosc Clin N Am 1995;5:587–93.
20. Wiersema MJ, Vilmann P, Giovannini M, et al. Endosonography-guided fine-needle aspiration biopsy; diagnostic accuracy and complication assessment. Gastroenterologist 1997;112:1087–95.
21. Vazquez-Sequerios E, Wiersema MJ, Clain JE, et al. Impact of lymph node staging on therapy of esophageal carcinoma. Gastroenterologist 2003;125: 1626–35.
22. Penman ID, Henry E. Advanced esophageal cancer. Gastrointest Endosc Clin N Am 2005;15:101–16.
23. Pfau PR, Ginsberg GG, Lew RJ, et al. EUS predictors of long-term survival in esophageal carcinoma. Gastrointest Endosc 2001;53:463–9.
24. Eloubeidi MA. Routine EUS-guided FNA for preoperative nodal staging in patients with esophageal carcinoma: is the juice worth the squeeze? Gastrointest Endosc 2006;63:212–4.
25. Jacobson BC, Chak A, Hoffman B, et al. Quality indicators for endoscopic ultrasonography. Am J Gastroenterol 2006;101:898–901.
26. Puli SR, Reddy JBK, Bechtold ML, et al. Accuracy of endoscopic ultrasound in the diagnosis of distal and celiac axis lymph node metastasis in esophageal cancer: a meta-analysis and systemic review. Dig Dis Sci 2008;53:2405–14.
27. Reed CE, Mishra G, Sahai AV, et al. Esophageal cancer staging: improved accuracy by endoscopic ultrasound of celiac lymph nodes. Ann Thorac Surg 1999;67: 319–21.
28. Christie NA, Rice TW, DeCamp MM, et al. M1a/M1b esophageal carcinoma: clinical relevance. J Thorac Cardiovasc Surg 1999;118:900–7.
29. Flamen P, Bourgeois S, Hiele M, et al. Positron emission tomography [PET] compared to EUS and spiral CT in staging of patients with potentially operable esophageal carcinoma. Gastroenterology 2000;118:256.
30. Nguyen P, Feng JC, Chang KJ. Endoscopic ultrasound (EUS) and EUS-guided fine-needle aspiration (FNA) of liver lesions. Gastrointest Endosc 1999;50:357–61.
31. McGrath K, Brody D, Luketich J, et al. Detection of unsuspected left hepatic lobe metastases during EUS staging of cancer of the esophagus and cardia. Am J Gastroenterol 2006;101:1742–6.
32. Prasad P, Schmulewitz N, Patel A, et al. Detection of occult liver metastases during EUS for staging of malignancies. Gastrointest Endosc 2004;1:49–53.
33. Saftoiu A, Vilmann P, Ciurea T, et al. Dynamic analysis of EUS used for the differentiation of benign and malignant lymph nodes. Gastrointest Endosc 2007;66: 291–300.
34. Saftoiu A, Vilman P. Endoscopic ultrasound elastography—a new imaging technique for the visualization of tissue elasticity distribution. J Gastrointestin Liver Dis 2006;15:161–5.
35. Dietrich CF. Comments and illustrations regarding the guidelines and good clinical practice recommendations for contrast-enhanced ultrasound (CEUS)—update 2008. Ultraschall Med 2008;29(Suppl 4):S188–202.

36. Salonen O, Kivisaari L, Standertskjold-Nordenstam C-G, et al. Computed tomography in staging of esophageal carcinoma. Scand J Gastroenterol 1987;22:65–8.
37. Halvorsen R, Magruder-Habib K, Foster W, et al. Esophageal cancer staging by CT: long-term follow-up study. Radiology 1986;161:147–51.
38. Tio TL, Cohen P, Coene PP, et al. Endosonography and computed tomography of esophageal carcinoma: preoperative classification compared to the new (1987) TNM system. Gastroenterology 1989;96:1478–86.
39. Chak A, Canto M, Gerdes H, et al. Prognosis of esophageal cancers preoperatively staged to be locally invasive (T4) by endoscopic ultrasound (EUS): a multicenter retrospective cohort study. Gastrointest Endosc 1995;42(6): 501–6.
40. Luketich JD, Friedman DM, Weigel TL, et al. Evaluation of distant metastases in esophageal cancer: 100 consecutive positron emission tomography scans. Ann Thorac Surg 1999;68:1133–6.
41. Lowe VJ, Booya F, Fletcher JG, et al. Comparison of positron emission tomography, computed tomography, and endoscopic ultrasound in the initial staging of patients with esophageal cancer. Mol Imaging Biol 2005;7:422–30.
42. McDonough PB, Jones DR, Shen KR, et al. Does FDG-PET add information to EUS and CT in the initial management of esophageal cancer? A prospective single center study. Am J Gastroenterol 2008;103:570–4.
43. Van Dam J, Rice TW, Catalano MF, et al. High-grade malignant stricture is predictive of esophageal tumor stage. Risks of endosonographic evaluation. Cancer 1993;71:2910–7.
44. Hiele M, De Leyn P, Schurmans P, et al. Relation between endoscopic ultrasound findings and outcome of patients with tumors of the esophagus or esophagogastric junction. Gastrointest Endosc 1997;45:381–6.
45. Catalano MF, Van Dam J, Sivak MV. Malignant esophageal strictures: staging accuracy of endoscopic ultrasonography. Gastrointest Endosc 1995;41:535–9.
46. Mallery S, Van Dam J. Increased rate of complete EUS staging of patients with esophageal cancer using the nonoptical, wire-guided echoendoscope. Gastrointest Endosc 1999;50:53–7.
47. Jacobson BC, Shami VM, Faigel DO, et al. Through-the-scope balloon dilation for endoscopic ultrasound staging of stenosing esophageal cancer. Dig Dis Sci 2007;52:817–22.
48. Kalha I, Kaw M, Fukami N, et al. The accuracy of endoscopic ultrasound for restaging esophageal carcinoma after chemoradiation therapy. Cancer 2004; 101(5):940–7.
49. Pfau PR, Chak A. Endoscopic ultrasonography. Endoscopy 2002;34:21–8.
50. Isenberg G, Chak A, Canto MI, et al. Endoscopic ultrasound in restaging of esophageal cancer after neoadjuvant chemoradiation. Gastrointest Endosc 1998;48:158–63.
51. Chak A, Canto MI, Cooper GS, et al. Endosonographic assessment of multimodality therapy predicts survival of esophageal carcinoma patients. Cancer 2000;88:1788–95.
52. Catalano MF, Sivak MV Jr, Rice TW, et al. Postoperative screening for anastomotic recurrence of esophageal carcinoma by endoscopic ultrasonography. Gastrointest Endosc 1995;42:540–4.
53. Fockens P, Manshanden CG, van Lanschot JJ, et al. Prospective study on the value of endosonographic follow-up after surgery for esophageal carcinoma. Gastrointest Endosc 1997;46:487–91.

The Role of FDG-PET and Staging Laparoscopy in the Management of Patients with Cancer of the Esophagus or Gastroesophageal Junction

Harry H. Yoon, MD, MHS[a],*, Val J. Lowe, MD[b],
Stephen D. Cassivi, MD, MSc[c], Yvonne Romero, MD[d,e]

KEYWORDS

- PET • CT • Esophageal cancer • Staging laparoscopy
- Treatment response • Staging
- Gastroesophageal junction cancer • Prognosis

Prognostically, esophageal cancer is characterized by high rates of local or distant recurrence following primary therapy, with death occurring soon after. Further darkening this grim prognosis is the observation that patients may spend their final months enduring and trying to recover from primary therapy, which often includes a potentially toxic combination of chemotherapy, radiation, and surgery.

The high failure rate is partly due to inadequacies in staging, which ideally would distinguish curable from incurable disease at the outset. Ideal staging selects patients for therapy according to the likelihood of clinical benefit—patients with local or locally advanced disease could receive local or multimodality therapy, whereas those with distant metastases could be spared aggressive and futile interventions.

[a] Division of Medical Oncology, Department of Oncology, Mayo Clinic, 200 First Street SW, Rochester, MN 55905, USA
[b] Division of Nuclear Medicine, Department of Radiology, Mayo Clinic, Rochester, MN 55906, USA
[c] Division of General Thoracic Surgery, Department of Surgery, Mayo Clinic, 200 First Street SW, Rochester, MN 55905, USA
[d] Division of Gastroenterology and Hepatology, Department of Medicine, Mayo Clinic, 200 First Street SW, Rochester, MN 55905, USA
[e] Department of Otolaryngology, Mayo Clinic, 200 First Street SW, Rochester, MN 55905, USA
* Corresponding author.
E-mail address: yoon.harry@mayo.edu (H.H. Yoon).

Gastroenterol Clin N Am 38 (2009) 105–120
doi:10.1016/j.gtc.2009.01.007
0889-8553/09/$ – see front matter © 2009 Elsevier Inc. All rights reserved.

For years, CT was the first-line method to detect distant metastases; however, major US trials enrolling patients thought to have resectable disease after CT with or without endoscopic ultrasonography (EUS) yielded noncurative resections in as many as 15% to 30% of patients and 1-year disease-free and overall survival rates of only 30% to 48% and 58% to 72%, respectively.[1,2] In recent years, CT has been reported to have a sensitivity and specificity for detecting distant metastases of 41% to 81% and 82% to 83%, respectively.[3,4]

When EUS was introduced, it became the most reliable method for determining T stage and identifying cancerous regional lymph nodes. EUS with fine-needle aspiration (FNA) enabled selective aspiration of echographically suspicious nodes, including those at the celiac axis; however, even when combined with CT, EUS has a reported sensitivity for detecting involved lymph nodes of only 11% to 54% and a specificity of 90% to 95%.[4] Moreover, EUS is limited in esophageal obstruction, which impedes adequate passage of the endoscope and accurate detection of the depth of invasion and metastatic disease.

While tremendous attention has focused on developing effective therapies in all stages of disease, another line of investigation has been to improve initial staging. Modalities that have received attention or become standard at some institutions include 2-deoxy-2-[^{18}F]fluoro-D-glucose positron emission tomography (FDG-PET) scanning, staging laparoscopy, and EUS.

PET has emerged as an important, increasingly common staging tool, particularly for the detection of distant metastases. Its routine use is recommended by the National Comprehensive Cancer Network in staging patients lacking M1 disease on CT and EUS. PET has also been studied to assess therapeutic response and to prognosticate, a role that is still investigational. Meanwhile, staging laparoscopy has been evaluated for the detection of peritoneal disease, particularly in patients with disease involving the gastroesophageal junction. Its acceptance has been less widespread. The role of EUS is discussed in detail elsewhere in this issue.

This article primarily reviews the data on the role of PET in staging and restaging esophageal cancer and in assessing the response to therapy. It also discusses the potential role of laparoscopy as a staging tool. Because of the dominance of adenocarcinoma in the United States and other Western countries, and because it appears to be a distinct clinical entity from squamous cell carcinoma, this discussion of the current literature draws attention to studies focusing on this histologic subtype.

POSITRON EMISSION TOMOGRAPHY IN INITIAL STAGING

CT and EUS provide anatomic visualization, whereas PET measures metabolic processes. PET can potentially determine quantitative information on blood flow, receptor status, and metabolic processes, depending on the radiopharmaceutical selected. Many of the early studies of PET in esophageal cancer were performed with "PET only" imaging. The advent of PET scanners with integrated CT scanners in recent years has allowed for direct comparison of metabolic information with anatomy with the added benefit of shorter imaging times for patients. This integration has led to an improvement in diagnostic accuracy from PET imaging; therefore, all state-of-the-art PET imaging is currently performed with integrated CT (PET/CT). The FDG is a glucose analogue that emits positron radiotracer. It is transported intracellularly and phosphorylated to FDG-6-phosphate via the same pathways as glucose. Because it is highly polarized, it is trapped in the cell. FDG-6-phosphate accumulates in tumors following injection and provides a signal of high glycolytic tissue activity in the body. Malignant tumors in most organ systems, except the brain and urinary tract, are frequently detected by FDG-PET.

PET images are analyzed qualitatively and quantitatively. The intensity of FDG uptake characterized as a standardized uptake value (SUV) within specific lesions is calculated as follows:

$$SUV = \frac{\text{mean activity in the region of interest}\,(mCi/mL)}{\text{injected dose of FDG}(mCi)/\text{body wt}(g)}$$

Assessing T Stage

PET/CT has limited use in T staging, although tumor invasion into adjacent organs (T4) can sometimes be detected. Signs of invasion into adjacent organs include blurring of periesophageal fat, loss of intervening fat planes, and a large concave interface.[5] After neoadjuvant radiotherapy, loss of normal tissue planes due to radiation-induced fibrosis and necrosis makes repeat evaluation of the T classification difficult with all imaging modalities, and local organ invasion may not be detected until esophagectomy.[5]

Key studies evaluating PET in the initial staging of patients with adenocarcinoma of the esophagus or gastroesophageal junction are shown in **Table 1**. The sensitivity of PET for detecting primary esophageal tumors has been reported in prospective studies to be 91% to 95%.[3,6] In one study of 75 esophageal cancer patients, PET correctly assessed T status in 43% of cases, understaged status in 29%, and over-staged status in 29%.[3] Given the limited spatial resolution of PET imaging devices (about 5–8 mm), it is generally believed that lesions smaller than 1 cm, particularly early stage cancers, may not be detected.

Assessing N Stage

Locoregional lymph nodes (eg, gastrohepatic ligament) are generally considered resectable (N1), whereas the resectability of celiac axis nodes is more controversial (M1a). Most studies indicate that PET, with or without CT, has limited use in assessing locoregional lymph node status (see **Table 1**). FDG uptake within periesophageal nodes close to the primary tumor is difficult to differentiate from uptake within the esophageal tumor itself due to the limited spatial resolution of PET. Further limiting the interpretation of nodes is the observation that FDG uptake can occur in benign disease such as granulomatous inflammation (eg, sarcoidosis), aspiration pneumonitis, or other inflammatory/infectious conditions.

A meta-analysis of 12 studies (n = 490) that examined the diagnostic accuracy of PET in preoperative staging of esophageal cancer reported sensitivity and specificity for detecting locoregional node involvement of 51% and 84%, respectively.[7] The studies in the meta-analysis were heterogeneous in methodologic quality, in whether preoperative EUS was incorporated, and in whether PET images were fused with images from CT.

A Belgian study[4] included in the meta-analysis reported the accuracy of PET in detecting local versus regional-distant nodal involvement (n = 74) and found accuracy rates to be similar between nodal regions. Local nodes were defined as those located within 3 cm from the primary tumor. Regional and distant nodes comprised all other nodes, including those in mediastinal, supraclavicular, and retroperitoneal areas. The sensitivity and specificity of PET were similar in the two nodal groups: 33% and 89% for local nodes and 46% and 90% for regional-distant nodes, respectively.

Subsequent to the meta-analysis, the authors reported the results of a prospective study at their institution comparing the accuracy of PET, CT, and EUS in the initial staging of patients with esophageal cancer (n = 75).[3] In contrast to other data, the

Table 1
Studies evaluating PET in initial staging of esophageal adenocarcinoma

Study	Institute	Design	Number of Patients	Other Modalities	AC/SCC (%)	T (%)[a]	N Sensitivity (%)	N Specificity (%)	M Sensitivity (%)	M Specificity (%)	PCM (%)
Block 1997[29]	Washington University	Unclear	58	CT	59/40	—[b]	—	—	—	—	15
Luketich 1997[30]	University of Pittsburgh	Retro	35	EUS, bscan, CT, Ls or Ts	71/26	97	45	100	88[c]	93[c]	20
Lowe 2005[3]	Mayo	Prosp	75	CT, EUS	90/10	—	82	60	81	91	4
Flamen 2000[4]	Gathuisberg, Belgium	Prosp	74	CT, EUS	72/28	95	39	97	74	90	—
Meyers 2007[6]	ACOSOG	Prosp	189	CT	NR	91	—	—	5%–10% Upstaged to M1b 3% Falsely upstaged to M1b		
Heeren 2004[10]	Groningen, Netherlands	Prosp	74	CT, EUS	84/16	95	55	71	78	98	7

Abbreviations: AC, adenocarcinoma; ACOSOG, American College of Surgeons Oncology Group; bscan, bone scan; EUS, endoscopic ultrasound; Ls, laparoscopy; M, metastasis; M1b, stage IV M1b denoting distant organ metastases; N, node; NR, not reported; PCM, PET changes management based on identification of M1b or otherwise unresectable disease missed by other modalities; Prosp, prospective; Retro, retrospective; SCC, squamous cell carcinoma; T, tumor; Ts, thoracoscopy.

[a] Sensitivity for identifying primary tumor. Specificity for detecting tumor was not assessed in most studies because inclusion criteria required the presence of primary esophageal tumor.

[b] Dash denotes results reported in a way that did not permit simple cross-study comparison.

[c] Distant metastases refers to M1b disease.

sensitivity of PET was found to be higher and the specificity of PET lower for detecting nodal metastases, that is, 82% and 60%, respectively.

Our reported specificity was probably lower because, unlike in other reports, EUS operators in the study were initially blinded to PET and CT results. After finishing TNM staging and sampling of visualized nodes, the EUS operator opened a sealed envelope to learn whether PET and CT had identified additional nodes or metastatic foci that could be assessed. If so, the operator sampled these areas, allowing histo-pathologic evaluation of all detected nodes in all modalities. Such pathologic confirmation could lead to a higher false-positivity rate (or lower specificity) attributed to PET or CT than reported elsewhere.

The sensitivity rate reported in our study was higher possibly because (1) we included both unresectable and resectable cases following CT evaluation, whereas other studies[8] excluded unresectable cases, and (2) we performed PET with attenuation correction, which is known to improve sensitivity.[9]

Changing Management: Evaluating Distant Disease (M Stage)

The crucial test for incorporating a diagnostic modality in staging work-up is the degree to which it rationally alters clinical management. In esophageal cancer, two anatomic-pathologic checkpoints can most affect clinical management. The first checkpoint is distinguishing T2 (submucosa) from T3 (serosa) lesions. T1-2 lesions may be cured with surgery alone, whereas T3 lesions are commonly managed with tri-modality therapy. As discussed previously, PET contributes minimally in this regard. The second checkpoint is distinguishing potentially resectable, locally advanced disease (T3-4N0, N1, perhaps M1a) from distant disease (M1b, perhaps M1a). Patients properly diagnosed with distant disease would receive more accurate prognostic information and palliative chemotherapy and would be spared combined chemoradiation and esophagectomy. For these patients, PET may be most helpful.

In their discussion, the investigators of the meta-analysis observed that patient management was altered in 3% to 20% cases due to the addition of PET in the preoperative work-up.[7] The large range is explained in part by differences in entry criteria, the rigor with which pathologic verification (gold standard) was obtained, the study design, and criteria for resectability.

In prospective studies with clear reporting and rigorous attempts at pathologic confirmation that distinguished between M1a and M1b disease, M1b disease was detected by PET and missed by CT (with or without EUS) in 5% to 7% of cases.[6,10] The addition of preoperative PET would have spared these patients unnecessary surgery.

One study reported that PET indicated M1b disease in an additional 10% of patients, but pathologic confirmation was not obtained.[6] The investigators clarified that these PET-avid M1b lesions were unlikely to be malignant, because many of the unconfirmed findings were noted in patients who subsequently underwent surgical resection and had no evidence of recurrence or progression at 6 months.

M1 disease of any type (M1a or M1b) was detected by PET and missed by CT (with or without EUS) in 6% to 15% of patients.[4,6,10] The minimal contribution of PET in detecting M1 disease in our study (1%) is perhaps explained by the fact that EUS detected M1a and some adjacent hepatic lesions with substantially greater sensitivity than reported elsewhere.[3,4,10]

Limitations and Risk of Positron Emission Tomography

A potential downside to the routine use of PET in staging is the burden imposed by false-positive findings. The specificity of PET for M1a or M1b disease has been reported consistently to be high (90%–98%).[3,4,7,10,11] Nevertheless, as with any diagnostic modality, false-positive findings lead to futile, potentially harmful work-up.

This problem is most aptly illustrated in the ACOSOG trial, one of few studies that reported adverse events stemming from the use of PET. In that trial, 4% of patients had negative confirmatory procedures. One patient underwent an adrenalectomy for a false-positive PET suggesting an adrenal metastasis. In addition to requiring a surgical procedure, the patient also required subsequent therapy for adrenal insufficiency. Another patient experienced a grade 3 adverse event for a wound complication after a confirmatory procedure for a false-positive finding.

REPEAT POSITRON EMISSION TOMOGRAPHY DURING OR AFTER NEOADJUVANT THERAPY AS A RESTAGING TOOL AND PROGNOSTIC MARKER

Based on the cumulative evidence of several underpowered trials, one standard therapy for resectable, locally advanced esophageal cancer in the United States has evolved to include chemotherapy concurrent with radiation (before surgery). Likewise, some parts of Europe have adopted neoadjuvant chemotherapy alone (followed by surgery). Both preoperative approaches have improved outcomes modestly at best and with considerable toxicity; therefore, investigators have sought ways to improve the selection of patients for therapy.

In this context the value of obtaining a repeat PET scan during or after neoadjuvant therapy has been studied as a restaging tool and as a prognostic marker. Three clinical scenarios have received the most attention in their potential for PET to alter and improve patient management (**Table 2**): (1) during neoadjuvant therapy for

Table 2
Rationale for obtaining repeat PET scan: three scenarios

Timing of Repeat PET	PET Features Assessed for Predictive Value	Outcomes Examined	Implication for Clinical Management
During neoadjuvant therapy	1. Change in FDG uptake (baseline versus repeat)	Pathologic response[a] or overall survival	Nonresponders:[b] alter chemotherapy agent or undergo immediate surgery Responders:[c] continue neoadjuvant chemo and subsequent surgery
After completion of neoadjuvant therapy, before potential surgery	2. Presence of unresectable disease in repeat PET scan	NA	Cancel surgery; palliative therapy
	3. Change in FDG uptake (baseline versus repeat)	Pathologic response[a] or overall survival	Nonresponders:[b] alter chemotherapy agent or undergo immediate surgery Responders:[c] forego or undergo surgery

Abbreviation: NA, not applicable.
[a] Assessed at surgery.
[b] Patient with persistent or progressive hypermetabolic activity on repeat PET scan.
[c] Patient with decreased hypermetabolic activity on repeat PET scan.

prognostication, (2) after neoadjuvant therapy and before surgery for restaging, and (3) after neoadjuvant therapy and before surgery for prognostication.

The scenario with the most straightforward implications is the use of PET after the completion of neoadjuvant therapy as a restaging tool before anticipated surgery (scenario two, see **Table 2**). Identifying the interval development of unresectable disease on repeat PET would disqualify the patient from surgery or other aggressive therapies. The treatment paradigm would shift to palliation. Because CT is commonly used to assess response, PET or PET/CT would need to add substantially to CT alone for integration after neoadjuvant therapy.

This particular question has not been extensively studied. One study prospectively enrolled 48 patients with esophageal cancer (85% adenocarcinoma) who were staged with CT, EUS-FNA, and PET/CT before and after neoadjuvant chemoradiation.[12] Patients with tissue confirmation of persistent nodal or metastatic disease who did not undergo complete resection were also included. Tissue biopsy was required to document M1b disease. Regarding the detection of M1b disease after chemoradiation, integrated PET/CT correctly identified four cases, falsely identified four cases, and missed two cases. CT performed similarly to PET/CT, correctly identifying three cases, falsely identifying three cases, and missing three cases. In this small study, PET/CT was superior to CT alone in finding evidence of distant disease, but at the price of a higher false-positive rate.

In another study, medical records were reviewed of patients scheduled to receive trimodality therapy who underwent PET/CT and esophagogastroduodenoscopy/ EUS at baseline and after neoadjuvant treatment.[13] Neoadjuvant therapy consisted of induction chemotherapy followed by chemoradiation, or chemoradiation alone. Among 88 patients who fit this profile, repeat PET/CT detected the interval development of M1b disease alone in three patients (3.4%). A fourth patient had M1a disease alone, and a fifth patient had both M1a and M1b disease. Of the three patients with M1b disease, two (2%) had metastases in skeletal muscle or bone marrow confirmed by biopsy or follow-up PET/CT. These disease sites are certainly outside the range of CT.

The sparse data that exist do not demonstrate substantial superiority of PET/CT over CT alone in the interval detection of unresectable disease after neoadjuvant therapy. In addition, one must consider the potential, albeit rare, risk of complications following confirmatory procedures, especially when the PET/CT abnormality may ultimately be deemed to reflect a false-positive finding. The use of PET/CT in this setting should not be considered mandatory until further data emerge. Balancing the substantial potential harm associated with an aborted esophagectomy due to metastases found at the time of laparotomy or, worse, a completed esophagectomy without survival benefit compared with the low likelihood of serious harm from pursuing a false-positive PET/CT abnormality, our multidisciplinary practice has increasingly employed PET/CT to detect the interval development of distant disease following neoadjuvant chemoradiation.

By contrast, a clinical time point that has been reported more extensively and with intriguing findings is the use of PET 2 to 3 weeks after initiating neoadjuvant therapy (scenario one, **Tables 2** and **3**). In a single-arm, single-institution study, a German group enrolled 65 patients with resectable, locally advanced adenocarcinoma of the gastroesophageal junction.[14] All patients were scheduled to receive chemotherapy alone followed by surgery. A PET scan was obtained at baseline and 2 weeks after the initiation of chemotherapy. Patients were classified as metabolic responders if the metabolic activity of the primary tumor had decreased by more than 35% at the time of the second PET and as nonresponders otherwise. Outcome variables were

Table 3
Studies evaluating metabolic response (repeat versus baseline PET) as prognostic marker in esophageal adenocarcinoma

Treatment Modality	Study	Institute	Number of Patients	Design	Timing of Repeat PET	Cutoff in SUV Decrease (%) to Denote Metabolic Responder	Pathologic Response[a]	Association Between Metabolic Response and Outcome (Responder Versus Nonresponder)			
								DFS or TTP		OS	
								UV (m)	MV (HR)	UV (m)	MV
C/S	Ott 2006[14]	Munich	65	Prosp, 1-arm	During[b]	>35	44% versus 5%	>42 versus 10	0.22	>32 versus 18	NS
	Port 2007[17]	Cornell	62	Retro	After[c]	>50	24% versus 4%	35 versus 18	2.4[d]	NR	NR
	Lordick 2007[31]	Munich	110	Prosp, 2-arm (PET guided)	During	>35	58% versus 0%	30 versus 14	NR	>27 versus 26	NR
CRT/S	Downey 2003[18]	MSKCC	24	Prosp, 1-arm	After	>60	NR	67% versus 38% (2 y) NS	NR	89% versus 63% (2 y) NS	NR
	Swisher 2004[32]	MD Anderson	83	Retro	After	Post-CRT SUV <4	—	NR	NR	60% versus 33% (2 y)	NR
C/CRT/S	Ribi 2007[19]	Swiss	56	Prosp, 1-arm	After C, before CRT	>40	—	NR	NR	NR	NR
	Ku 2007[20]	MSKCC	55	Prosp, 1-arm	After C, before CRT	>35	—	41 versus 9	NR	HR 0.9	NR

Abbreviations: C/S, chemotherapy followed by surgery; CRT/S, chemoradiation followed by surgery; C/CRT/S, induction chemotherapy followed by chemoradiation followed by surgery; DFS, disease-free survival; HR, hazard ratio for death; m, months (median); MSKCC, Memorial Sloan Kettering Cancer Center; MV, multivariate; NA, not applicable; NR, not reported; NS, statistically nonsignificant at alpha 0.05; OS, overall survival; Prosp, prospective; Retro, retrospective; TTP, time to progression; UV, univariate; y, year.

[a] Percent of patients with absence, near absence, or with presumed decrease of tumor cells in resected specimen.

[b] During neoadjuvant therapy.

[c] Following the completion of neoadjuvant therapy.

[d] HR for death comparing nonresponder with responder statistically significant at alpha 0.05.

the presence of a histopathologic "response" (ie, less than 10% tumor cells in the resected specimen) and overall survival.

Nine patients were excluded because baseline FDG uptake was too low (n = 8) or blood glucose was too high at repeat PET (n = 1). Of the remaining 56 patients, 6 experienced disease progression and the other 50 reached surgery. Of the 50, 41 patients underwent surgery with cancer-free margins.

The investigators found that metabolic responders when compared with nonresponders were more likely to have a histopathologic response (44% versus 5%, P = .001) and to live longer (3-year overall survival rate of 70% versus 35%, P = .01). Furthermore, multivariate modeling revealed that a metabolic response predicted risk independently (hazard ratio [HR] for death, 0.34, when comparing responders with nonresponders). This finding held true when limiting analysis to patients who reached operation. It also held true when assessing disease-free survival among patients with cancer-free resection margins.

Although these results are intriguing and warrant further testing, they should be interpreted with caution in their clinical implementation. First, simple associations with outcome are insufficient evidence to rationally affect clinical management. What is necessary are predictive values or likelihood ratios followed by validation studies. The investigators reported positive and negative predictive values with regard to histopathologic response and clinical response. The former is perhaps the strongest prognosticator of overall outcome, but neither factor has been demonstrated to be a valid surrogate of meaningful clinical outcome. Overall survival was not assessed with regard to PET findings.

Second, subjects in the study may be highly selected and not reflect those in the general population. The median survival in this cohort far exceeded that reported in patients in the combined chemotherapy/surgery arms of large randomized trials (32 versus 15–17 months).[1,15] One can speculate that survival in the general population is worse.

Third, the generalizability of the findings is further limited because 14% of subjects enrolled were excluded from analysis, mostly due to insufficient uptake on their baseline PET.

Fourth, further diminishing generalizability is the fact that treatment consisted of chemotherapy alone and not chemoradiation. Metabolic response and PET interpretation (eg, determining threshold cutoff values) may differ between patients who receive chemotherapy versus chemoradiation.

Lastly and perhaps most problematic is the fact that, without a randomized trial, the appropriate triage of nonresponders (or responders) is unknown. It has been suggested that nonresponders be sent down a variety of therapeutic paths, all mutually exclusive, as follows: (1) immediate surgery (under the rationale that chemotherapy adds only modest benefit to surgery anyway, and for nonresponders will only add toxicity), (2) palliation alone (under the rationale that neither chemotherapy nor surgery will help), or (3) the use of a new chemotherapy agent followed by surgery (under the rationale that surgery alone has been demonstrated to have poor outcomes and that response to a new agent may be better).

To clarify these issues, a randomized phase II trial (MUNICON) was led by the same German group. Patients with locally advanced gastroesophageal cancer (n = 119) were enrolled to assess the metabolic response as a means to guide subsequent therapy. PET was obtained at baseline and after 2 weeks of chemotherapy. Metabolic responders (using a >35% decrease in SUV as the cutoff) continued with chemotherapy and then underwent surgery. Nonresponders discontinued chemotherapy and underwent immediate surgery. One hundred ten patients were evaluable for metabolic response, half of whom were responders. Patients were followed up for a mean of 2.3 years.

The most important finding was that the overall survival of nonresponders (26 months) who were denied chemotherapy did not appear to be lower than that of historical controls who received chemotherapy and surgery (15–18 months).[1,14,15] Nevertheless, again, the cohort as a whole appears to have been highly selected, because their overall survival exceeded that in other trials.

In addition, the correct allocation of responders or nonresponders is still unknown. Whether responders would perform just as well without further chemotherapy, and whether nonresponders would have performed better with further chemotherapy remain unanswered. Until these questions are addressed in a randomized trial, assessing the PET response during induction therapy should be considered investigational.

Assessing treatment response by PET has also been studied following the completion of neoadjuvant therapy (scenario three, see **Tables 2** and **3**). The outcomes that PET has been assessed against include the pathologic response (ie, complete absence versus residual tumor in the resected specimen) and the disease-free or overall survival.

PET has been consistently demonstrated to be unreliable in predicting a pathologic complete response (pCR) after neoadjuvant chemotherapy or chemoradiation. One group retrospectively reviewed the records of patients who underwent trimodality therapy and who had PET between chemoradiation and surgery.[16] Among 19 patients whose tumor was more PET avid than adjacent irradiated esophagus, suggesting residual disease, at least five had a pCR. Furthermore, among 23 patients whose tumor was less PET avid than adjacent irradiated esophagus, suggesting tumor clearance, 16 had residual (mostly microscopic) tumor.

Another study reviewed the records of patients who received neoadjuvant chemotherapy alone followed by surgery, with similar results.[17] Among 13 patients who had a 100% reduction in their SUV after chemotherapy, suggesting tumor clearance, only two had a pCR. The other patients had gross (n = 8) or microscopic (n = 3) residual disease. A third study found that the positive predictive value of PET/CT for identifying a pCR was 76%, statistically similar to that found by CT (57%) or EUS-FNA (60%).

The link between metabolic response and survival has also been evaluated, often generating positive associations of important scientific interest and limited or unclear clinical relevance. One group reviewed the records of patients (n = 83, mostly adenocarcinoma) who received chemoradiation therapy followed by surgery, with CT, EUS, and PET performed before and after chemoradiation. After chemoradiotherapy, an SUV of four or greater on PET was the only preoperative factor that correlated with decreased survival (2-year survival rate of 33% versus 60%, P = .01). Multivariate analysis was not reported. In another single-institution study, a prospective study, metabolic responders had improved disease-free (67% versus 38%) and overall (89% versus 63%) survival at 2 years when compared with nonresponders.[18] Whether metabolic response was an independent predictor of outcome was not reported.

By themselves, these results do not clarify how to manage metabolic responders versus nonresponders following chemoradiation, for the same reasons it is unclear how to manage responders versus nonresponders after chemotherapy alone. We do not believe PET should be used routinely to assess the response after chemoradiation for guiding subsequent therapy. For now, the major clinical role of PET following neoadjuvant chemoradiation therapy remains the identification of distant metastases before performing esophagectomy.

Preliminary studies such as these open the way for further protocols to explore these questions, much as the MUNICON study has done. The effort to improve complete pathologic responses has led to trials in which chemoradiation and surgery are preceded by induction chemotherapy. Appropriately, studies have begun to assess the role of PET in these therapeutic contexts as well.[19,20]

STAGING LAPAROSCOPY

Minimally invasive surgery, including laparoscopy with or without thoracoscopy, has been proposed as a way of improving staging and has yielded reports of its diagnostic superiority over EUS or CT (**Table 4**).[11,21–27] Laparoscopic staging typically involves direct visualization and biopsy of abnormal findings on the peritoneal and liver surfaces. Entry into the lesser sac by incising the gastrohepatic ligament allows for potential sampling of lymph nodes adjacent to the lesser curve and celiac axis (lymph node stations 16–20).

The main potential benefit of staging laparoscopy is its ability to detect distant metastases missed by conventional imaging, thereby protecting the patient from a meaningless laparotomy. In addition, laparoscopy allows pathologic confirmation of nodal status, which could aid prognostication, help define radiation fields, and allocate unimodality versus trimodality therapy. Proponents of staging laparoscopy have pointed to other benefits, including better assessment of primary tumor size;[23] providing tissue samples to assess the prognostic ability of molecular markers;[25] the fact that staging laparoscopy, unlike EUS, is not prevented or limited by esophageal obstruction; and the possibility for inserting an enteral feeding tube before the stresses of anticipated chemoradiation.

Single-institution experience indicates that laparoscopy, when CT and EUS are used, substantially increases the sensitivity and specificity for detecting lymph node and distant metastases. Following CT and EUS, laparoscopy upstages nodal status in 0% to 21%[22–25] of cases and downstages in 4% to 19%.[22,24,25] Moreover, laparoscopy detects liver or peritoneal metastases in 7% to 20% of patients,[22–25] in which case the therapeutic paradigm is altered toward palliation. In one series (n = 59), staging laparoscopy following CT and EUS changed the tumor diagnosis in six patients from esophageal to gastric cancer.[22] Four patients with localized gastric cancer underwent gastrectomy, whereas two with advanced disease, that was otherwise occult, were treated with palliative measures only.

In the largest series to date (n = 511) of esophageal and gastric cancer patients, staging laparoscopy changed treatment primarily in patients with disease located in the lower esophagus or proximal stomach and never in the upper or mid esophagus. A major weakness of this study is that less than 10% patients (48/511) received both EUS and CT. A multicenter trial (CALGB 9380) was performed to evaluate the accuracy of staging laparoscopy, but it too was limited in that only half the patients underwent baseline EUS.[26] Follow-up data for that trial have not been reported (M.J. Krasna, personal communication, 2008).[28]

Major complications have been reported in 0% to 4%[22,23,25,26] of cases, with no reported mortality. In one series (n = 59)[22] in which feeding tubes were placed, one patient had a perforation of the small bowel adjacent to the J-tube insertion site and required laparotomy with small bowel resection. A second patient experienced intraoperative pulmonary edema secondary to unexpected aortic valve stenosis, which eventually required an aortic valve replacement before esophagectomy. An older series (n = 26) reported prolonged ileus (n = 2), atelectasis (2), urinary retention (2), port site infection (2), and small bowel obstruction (1).[11] Mean hospital stays lasted 2 to 3 days.[11,22,23,26]

Table 4
Studies assessing staging laparoscopy in esophageal cancer[a]

Study	Institution	Number of Patients	Design	Results				
				N (% up, down)	M (% up, down)	Management Change (%)[b]	Days in Hospital	Complications (%)[c]
Krasna 2002	University of Maryland[25]	76	Prosp	21, 9	7, —[d]	NR	NR	0
Kaiser 2007	Essen, Germany[23]	70	Retro	17, —	20, 0	20	3	0
Kaushik 2007	Pittsburgh[24]	47	Retro	0, 4	17, 6	—	NR	NR
Krasna 2001	CALGB[26]	113	Prosp	14, NR	2, NR	NR	3	0
Heath 2000	Hopkins[22]	59	Prosp	2, 19	≥7, NR	17	2	3
deGraaf 2007[e]	Nottingham, England[21]	416	Retro	—	—	20	NR	0
Luketich 1993[f]	Pittsburgh[11]	26	Prosp	11, 1	4, —	—	1.8	1

Abbreviations: Down, downstaged after laparoscopy; M, metastatic stage; N, nodal stage; NR, not reported for esophageal cancer or laparoscopy specifically; Pro, prospective; Retro, retrospective; Up, upstaged after laparoscopy.

[a] All studies except Krasna, 2001[26] and deGraaf, 2007[21] performed CT and endoscopic ultrasound in more than 70% of patients before laparoscopy.
[b] Results of staging laparoscopy changed clinical management.
[c] "Major" complication due to laparoscopy.
[d] Dash denotes results that were unclearly reported or did not permit simple cross-study comparison.
[e] Includes noncardia gastric cancer patients.
[f] Thoracoscopy performed with laparoscopy.

To date, in all reported series assessing staging laparoscopy, PET has not been included in the staging algorithm. This absence substantially limits the generalizability of the reports, because PET has reasonable accuracy for the detection of distant metastases[7] and has become a mainstay in the staging work-up of esophageal cancer.

It is unclear whether PET would have accurately detected the metastases discovered by laparoscopy in the previous series, because the sizes of those lesions were usually not reported. Notably, one prospective study (n = 74) in which therapy consisted of surgery alone found that peritoneal carcinomatosis was missed in five patients (6.7%) by both CT and PET and was discovered only at the time of laparotomy.[10] Whether this lack of sensitivity would have altered management depends on the surgical practice, because four of these patients also had PET-avid celiac or para-aortic nodes before surgery, which would have precluded resection in some centers.

Some investigators who appear to favor staging laparoscopy have acknowledged that the standard use of PET limits the role of laparoscopy to situations in which PET, CT, and EUS fail or are not feasible. Such situations would include that of a suspicious lymph node that is either inaccessible for biopsy or yields a negative or ambiguous pathologic reading on FNA.[26]

Furthermore, a cost-effectiveness analysis evaluating CT, EUS-FNA, PET, thoracoscopy/laparoscopy, and combinations thereof found that CT plus EUS-FNA was the least expensive strategy and offered more quality-adjusted life-years than all other strategies with the exception of PET plus EUS-FNA.[28] The latter was slightly more effective but more expensive. The investigators recommend PET plus EUS-FNA as the staging procedure for patients with esophageal cancer unless resources are scarce or PET is unavailable.

At the authors' center, EUS-FNA and integrated PET/CT are incorporated as the standard in the initial staging of all patients with esophageal cancer. We initially use a dedicated CT scan of the chest and abdomen because of its better anatomic definition to evaluate the extent of local invasion and screen for distant metastases. If none are found, PET/CT is used for further evaluation. If distant metastases are suggested by these imaging modalities, tissue confirmation is obtained. Only in cases in which no distant disease is suspected and curative resection remains a treatment option do we pursue EUS-FNA. Laparoscopy and thoracoscopy are reserved for situations in which the findings from history, physical examination, EUS-FNA, or PET/CT are equivocal and evidence of M1b disease would alter the planned treatment. Laparoscopy for staging is also performed at the time of placement of a laparoscopic feeding jejunostomy if one is required before esophagectomy. In the PET/CT era, we have not yet found a sufficient diagnostic or prognostic benefit for the patient to support the routine addition of laparoscopy in the staging of esophageal cancer.

SUMMARY

At the authors' center, patients with biopsy-proven submucosally invasive cancer of the esophagus or gastroesophageal junction routinely undergo the following staging work-up: CT of the chest and abdomen, integrated PET/CT scan and EUS-FNA, and other testing targeted to specific findings elicited on the history and physical examination. We do not perform routine staging laparoscopy or thoracoscopy and reserve these modalities for specific situations in which the testing results are equivocal and different findings would alter the treatment options. Localized early stage esophageal cancer is treated with esophagectomy alone, whereas locally advanced resectable disease is treated by neoadjuvant chemoradiation followed by surgery. Following chemoradiation, repeat CT is performed to identify interval development of unresectable disease. Among our oncology providers, the use of PET/CT to detect the interval development of distant disease is currently physician dependent. At present, the use of PET/CT to assess treatment response and influence subsequent therapy is investigational.

REFERENCES

1. Kelsen DP, Ginsberg R, Pajak TF, et al. Chemotherapy followed by surgery compared with surgery alone for localized esophageal cancer. N Engl J Med 1998;339(27):1979–84.
2. Urba SG, Orringer MB, Turrisi A, et al. Randomized trial of preoperative chemoradiation versus surgery alone in patients with locoregional esophageal carcinoma. J Clin Oncol 2001;19(2):305–13.
3. Lowe VJ, Booya F, Fletcher JG, et al. Comparison of positron emission tomography, computed tomography, and endoscopic ultrasound in the initial staging of patients with esophageal cancer. Mol Imaging Biol 2005;7(6):422–30.
4. Flamen P, Lerut A, Van Cutsem E, et al. Utility of positron emission tomography for the staging of patients with potentially operable esophageal carcinoma. J Clin Oncol 2000;18(18):3202–10.
5. Bruzzi JF, Munden RF, Truong MT, et al. PET/CT of esophageal cancer: its role in clinical management. Radiographics 2007;27(6):1635–52.
6. Meyers BF, Downey RJ, Decker PA, et al. The utility of positron emission tomography in staging of potentially operable carcinoma of the thoracic esophagus: results of the American College of Surgeons Oncology Group Z0060 trial. J Thorac Cardiovasc Surg 2007;133(3):738–45.
7. van Westreenen HL, Westerterp M, Bossuyt PM, et al. Systematic review of the staging performance of 18F-fluorodeoxyglucose positron emission tomography in esophageal cancer. J Clin Oncol 2004;22(18):3805–12.
8. Kneist W, Schreckenberger M, Bartenstein P, et al. Positron emission tomography for staging esophageal cancer: does it lead to a different therapeutic approach? World J Surg 2003;27(10):1105–12.
9. Rice TW. Clinical staging of esophageal carcinoma: CT, EUS, and PET. Chest Surg Clin N Am 2000;10(3):471–85.
10. Heeren PA, Jager PL, Bongaerts F, et al. Detection of distant metastases in esophageal cancer with (18)F-FDG PET. J Nucl Med 2004;45(6):980–7.
11. Luketich JD, Schauer P, Landreneau R, et al. Minimally invasive surgical staging is superior to endoscopic ultrasound in detecting lymph node metastases in esophageal cancer. J Thorac Cardiovasc Surg 1997;114(5):817–21 [discussion: 21–3].
12. Cerfolio RJ, Bryant AS, Ohja B, et al. The accuracy of endoscopic ultrasonography with fine-needle aspiration, integrated positron emission tomography with computed tomography, and computed tomography in restaging patients with esophageal cancer after neoadjuvant chemoradiotherapy. J Thorac Cardiovasc Surg 2005;129(6):1232–41.
13. Bruzzi JF, Swisher SG, Truong MT, et al. Detection of interval distant metastases: clinical utility of integrated CT-PET imaging in patients with esophageal carcinoma after neoadjuvant therapy. Cancer 2007;109(1):125–34.
14. Ott K, Weber WA, Lordick F, et al. Metabolic imaging predicts response, survival, and recurrence in adenocarcinomas of the esophagogastric junction. J Clin Oncol 2006;24(29):4692–8.

15. Medical Research Council Oesophageal Cancer Working Party. Surgical resection with or without preoperative chemotherapy in oesophageal cancer: a randomised controlled trial. Lancet 2002;359(9319):1727–33.
16. Erasmus JJ, Munden RF, Truong MT, et al. Preoperative chemoradiation-induced ulceration in patients with esophageal cancer: a confounding factor in tumor response assessment in integrated computed tomographic-positron emission tomographic imaging. J Thorac Oncol 2006;1(5):478–86.
17. Port JL, Lee PC, Korst RJ, et al. Positron emission tomographic scanning predicts survival after induction chemotherapy for esophageal carcinoma. Ann Thorac Surg 2007;84(2):393–400.
18. Downey RJ, Akhurst T, Ilson D, et al. Whole body [18]FDG-PET and the response of esophageal cancer to induction therapy: results of a prospective trial. J Clin Oncol 2003;21(3):428–32.
19. Ribi K, Nitzsche E, Schuller J, et al. PET scanning and patient reported dysphagia before and after chemotherapy (CT) for prediction of pathological response after CT and chemoradiotherapy (CRT) in patients with locally advanced esophageal cancer (EC): a multicenter phase II trial of the Swiss. 2007 ASCO Annual Meeting Proceedings Part I. Journal of Clinical Oncology 2007; 25(June 20 Supplement):4587.
20. Gea KU. Phase II trial of preoperative cisplatin/irinotecan and radiotherapy for locally advanced esophageal cancer: PET scan after induction therapy may identify early treatment failure. ASCO Gastrointestinal Cancers Symposium 2007. Available at: http://www.asco.org/ASCO/Abstracts+%26+Virtual+Meeting/Abstracts?&vmview=abst_detail_view&confID=45&abstractID=10131. Accessed September 23, 2008.
21. de Graaf GW, Ayantunde AA, Parsons SL, et al. The role of staging laparoscopy in oesophagogastric cancers. Eur J Surg Oncol 2007;33(8):988–92.
22. Heath EI, Kaufman HS, Talamini MA, et al. The role of laparoscopy in preoperative staging of esophageal cancer. Surg Endosc 2000;14(5):495–9.
23. Kaiser GM, Sotiropoulos GC, Fruhauf NR, et al. Value of staging laparoscopy for multimodal therapy planning in esophagogastric cancer. Int Surg 2007;92(3):128–32.
24. Kaushik N, Khalid A, Brody D, et al. Endoscopic ultrasound compared with laparoscopy for staging esophageal cancer. Ann Thorac Surg 2007;83(6): 2000–2.
25. Krasna MJ, Jiao X, Mao YS, et al. Thoracoscopy/laparoscopy in the staging of esophageal cancer: Maryland experience. Surg Laparosc Endosc Percutan Tech 2002;12(4):213–8.
26. Krasna MJ, Reed CE, Nedzwiecki D, et al. CALGB 9380: a prospective trial of the feasibility of thoracoscopy/laparoscopy in staging esophageal cancer. Ann Thorac Surg 2001;71(4):1073–9.
27. Patel AN, Buenaventura PO. Current staging of esophageal carcinoma. Surg Clin North Am 2005;85(3):555–67.
28. Wallace MB, Nietert PJ, Earle C, et al. An analysis of multiple staging management strategies for carcinoma of the esophagus: computed tomography, endoscopic ultrasound, positron emission tomography, and thoracoscopy/laparoscopy. Ann Thorac Surg 2002;74(4):1026–32.
29. Block M, Patterson GA, Sundaresan RS, et al. Improvement in staging of esophageal cancer with the addition of positron emission tomography. Ann Thorac Surg 1997;64:770–7.
30. Luketich JD, Schauer PR, Meltzer CC, et al. Role of positron emission tomography in staging esophageal cancer. Ann Thorac Surg 1997;64(3):765–9.

31. Lordick F, Ott K, Krause BJ, et al. PET to assess early metabolic response and to guide treatment of adenocarcinoma of the oesophagogastric junction: the MUNICON phase II trial. Lancet Oncol 2007;8(9):797–805.
32. Swisher SG, Erasmus J, Maish M, et al. 2-Fluoro-2-deoxy-D-glucose positron emission tomography imaging is predictive of pathologic response and survival after preoperative chemoradiation in patients with esophageal carcinoma. Cancer 2004;101(8):1776–85.

New Treatments, New Challenges: Pathology's Perspective on Esophageal Carcinoma

Jennifer R. Scudiere, MD, Elizabeth A. Montgomery, MD*

KEYWORDS

- Esophagus • Carcinoma • Duplication • Barrett
- Treatment • Prognosis

In 2008, an estimated 16,470 people in the United States were told that they have esophageal carcinoma.[1] During the same year, an estimated 14,280 people died of this disease.[1] This high rate of mortality occurs even though the esophagus is in a relatively accessible location and the use of screening endoscopy is widespread. One reason for the high mortality is the difficulty in properly identifying and treating early lesions. While frank esophageal carcinoma rarely presents a diagnostic challenge, early lesions are often tricky to address. Classification systems designed to stratify early lesions to make treatment decisions are complex and wrought with specific pathologic challenges brought on by new treatment modalities. Such interventions as endoscopic mucosal resection, photodynamic therapy, and chemotherapy/radiation combinations present the pathologist with new histologic challenges that have direct impact on patient care. In this article, we discuss staging issues pertinent to early cancers, histologic sequelae of various treatments, and how these factors affect the pathologist's role in evaluating esophageal carcinoma.

While the esophagus can harbor a range of neoplasms, two major types of primary esophageal carcinoma comprise the bulk of epithelial lesions in this location: squamous carcinoma and adenocarcinoma. Surveillance endoscopy is particularly useful in the evaluation of columnar lesions because it is practical and reliable for identifying and following, via biopsy, Barrett mucosa, a well-established precursor lesion.[2] While patients diagnosed with a deeply invasive carcinoma are usually treated with chemotherapy and radiation followed by surgery, many patients with early lesions are today

Department of Pathology, The Johns Hopkins Medical Institutions, The Harry and Jeanette Weinberg Building, 401 N. Broadway Room 2242, Baltimore, MD 21231-2410, USA
* Corresponding author.
E-mail address: emontgom@jhmi.edu (E.A. Montgomery).

Gastroenterol Clin N Am 38 (2009) 121–133
doi:10.1016/j.gtc.2009.01.011
0889-8553/09/$ – see front matter © 2009 Elsevier Inc. All rights reserved.

gastro.theclinics.com

managed endoscopically. As Heisenberg notes, the act of observation itself changes the entity observed. In the case of esophageal surveillance, the physician does more than just observe; the physician also takes multiple biopsies to evaluate the areas in question. While some changes are seen in Barrett mucosa before medical intervention (eg, duplication of the muscularis mucosae, discussed in the following pages), other changes are created iatrogenically as therapeutic measures or as side effects of these therapeutic measures.

CHANGES ASSOCIATED WITH BARRETT ESOPHAGUS: REDUPLICATION OF THE MUSCULARIS MUCOSAE AND IMPLICATIONS FOR STAGING

One of the most important recent advances in the evaluation of early esophageal lesions is the recognition and documentation of features of Barrett mucosa beyond the simple presence of intestinal metaplasia. The first mention of such additional features of Barrett mucosa was Rubio and Riddell's description[3] of the "musculo-fibrous anomaly" in Barrett esophagus. In this and a subsequent study, Rubio and Riddell[3,4] noted specific changes in the muscularis mucosae, lamina propria, and submucosa, as well as in the epithelium, in association with approximately 81% of Barrett esophagus patients evaluated. These evaluations paved the way for additional observations that led to the description of muscularis mucosae duplication in 1990.[5] In subsequent years, reports were published that substantiated and expanded on these findings.[6,7] Barrett esophagus came to be recognized as more than just an epithelial lesion; it blossomed into an entity that encompassed the lamina propria, muscularis mucosae, and even the submucosa. The feature that arguably creates the most diagnostic difficulty for the pathologist is the formation of multiple muscularis mucosae layers. In areas of intestinal metaplasia, two (or more) layers of muscularis mucosae can be seen. Often these muscular layers are not well delineated, and sparse wisps of muscle are seen between the layers with intermixed loose lamina propria tissue (**Fig. 1**). The deeper muscularis layer is generally recognized as the original layer, and the superficial layer (the layer closest to the luminal surface) is regarded as the "new" layer.[8,9] This designation is accepted in part because a direct connection between the deepest layer and the muscularis mucosae in adjacent non-Barrett esophagus can often be identified.

Surprisingly, however, once the phenomenon of muscularis mucosae duplication was recognized and accepted, it was largely ignored in the subsequent literature until recently.[10] Even as investigators fashioned increasingly detailed methods of subclassifying early lesions, muscularis mucosae duplication was not addressed, creating a particularly confounding situation for pathologists facing increasing numbers of endoscopic mucosal resection specimens.[10–12] Muscularis mucosae duplication and related changes, in addition to intestinal metaplasia, in Barrett esophagus occur in approximately 90% of resection specimens.[6–8,10] With such an overwhelming majority of specimens harboring these changes, a clear consensus regarding pathologic staging of adenocarcinomas is essential in the evaluation of specimens for treatment planning and prognostic purposes. Muscularis mucosae duplication remains incompletely understood.

The dilemma for pathologists arises when early adenocarcinoma is detected in a specimen that harbors muscularis mucosae duplication in the setting of Barrett esophagus. The classification of tumor depth for superficial esophageal cancer was first developed for squamous rather than columnar lesions by Japanese colleagues[13] and is described in **Fig. 2**. This classification is difficult to apply in the setting of duplicated muscularis mucosae, however. When the carcinoma extends to a portion of the

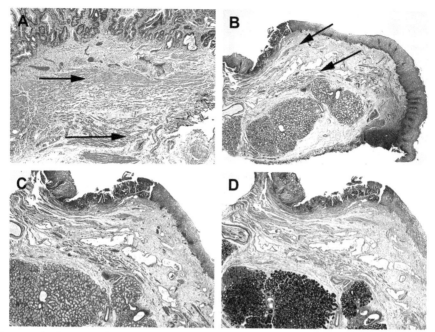

Fig. 1. Reduplication of the muscularis mucosae. (*A*) Two layers of muscularis mucosae are seen in this endoscopic mucosal resection specimen of Barrett esophagus (*arrows*). (*B*) Low-power view of an endoscopic mucosal resection specimen showing muscularis mucosae duplication beneath an area of Barrett esophagus with dysplasia. Arrows indicate muscularis mucosae layers. (*C*) A higher-power view of the same specimen as in B. (*D*) Periodic acid-Schiff/alcian-blue stain of the same specimen shown in B and C. This stain highlights the submucosal esophageal glands (*lower left portion of the field*), which are consistently alcianophilic. The submucosal glands are often useful for identification of the true submucosa in the setting of muscularis mucosae duplication.

muscularis mucosae or the area between duplicated muscularis mucosae layers, the pathologist must choose to classify the lesion as either an M3 lesion (T1a) or a submucosal lesion (T1b). The dilemma is illustrated in **Fig. 3**. That figure shows the carcinoma extending to the area between the two (or more) layers of muscularis mucosae (*arrows*). It remains controversial as to whether this area of lamina propria "between" muscularis mucosae layers is best interpreted as submucosa (since it is beyond some muscularis mucosae), or muscularis mucosae itself (since it has not extended beyond both muscularis mucosae). In interpreting superficial or tangentially embedded samples, the pathologist risks identifying the original (or deepest) layer of muscularis mucosae as muscularis propria, thereby mistaking a T1 lesion for a T2 lesion.

Assigning these criteria is not useful unless there are evidenced-based reasons to choose specific therapy based on the assignments. To this end, Hahn and colleagues[8] evaluated the composition of vascular constituents in both the superficial and deep lamina proprias in 30 patients undergoing esophagogastrectomy, 24 of which had Barrett esophagus. In this series, the density of blood and lymphatic vessels (as identified by CD31 and D2-40 expression, respectively, by immunohistochemistry) did not significantly differ in the submucosal tissue of Barrett esophagus (superficial as well as deep components when duplication occurred) compared with the submucosal tissues of the non-metaplastic squamous esophagus. The investigators concluded that the

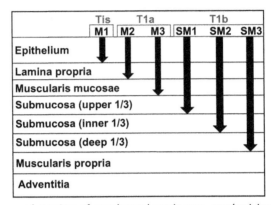

Fig. 2. Classification and staging of esophageal carcinoma, emphasizing early lesions. The arrows correspond to tumor depth. When lesional cells remain in the epithelium, the lesion is regarded as Tis or in situ, with a depth of M1. When the lesional cells extend into but not through the lamina propria, the lesion is designated T1a M2. Only early lesions (those that do not extend into the muscularis propria) are classified in this manner (up to T1b).

duplicated (or "new") muscularis mucosae simply separates the lamina propria into two compartments that do not differ substantially in their vascular constitutents, and should therefore be considered as one lamina propria for purposes of staging,[8] an assertion that remains unvalidated with long-term follow-up studies. It is not yet clear whether or not the "superficial" or "deep" lamina proprias created by the duplicated muscularis mucosae should be considered distinct staging locations under the rubric of intramucosal carcinoma.

Because tumor stage is such an important prognostic indicator, there is great interest in developing a staging system that best represents current knowledge. The current TNM staging system was developed by Pierre Denoix between 1943 and 1952, and has undergone multiple modifications throughout the years to reflect changing knowledge.[14,15] In a nutshell, the TNM staging system evaluates a particular patient's disease by assessing the tumor size and spread, the number and location of lymph nodes involved, and the presence and location of metastatic disease. After

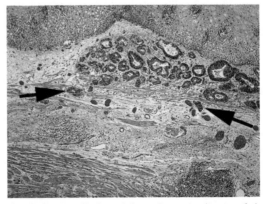

Fig. 3. The clusters of neoplastic cells (*arrows*) are between layers of duplicated muscularis mucosae. Current knowledge suggests that this lesion is best classified as an M3 (T1a) lesion.

categories are assigned for T, N, and M, a stage is assigned based on a chart, with stages ranging from stage 0 to stage IVB. Rolling modifications to the TNM system are an expected result of growing medical knowledge. The system has evolved along with medical technology, and has changed over the years to represent a more inter-disciplinary approach to disease as opposed to a clinician-centric or pathologist-centric classification system. Before 1987, the classification system had different criteria for pathologic staging of T1 and T2 esophageal lesions, with the clinical defi-nition depending on tumor surface area and the pathologic definition depending on invasion depth.[15] Today, proposals for the modification of the TNM staging system can be submitted to the International Union Against Cancer (http://www.uicc.org). Each proposal must include a rationale, analyses of the study, validation of the study, and specific recommendations for classification revision. In the most widely used international staging systems today, lesions invading the lamina and submucosa are both "lumped" as T1, which clearly is misleading for those patients whose lesions are restricted to the lamina propria, as those patients enjoy a better prognosis.

In the past few years, there has been an outcry to further modify the TNM staging system for esophageal carcinoma to better reflect evident patient outcomes. It is widely believed that the sixth edition of the International Union Against Cancer TNM guidelines for staging esophageal carcinoma could usefully be supplemented with additional tumor characteristics to focus on the patients' prognosis. In 2003, Rice and colleagues[16] evaluated 480 patients who underwent esophagectomy and concluded that the American Joint Committee on Cancer staging of esophageal cancer needed modifications to better reflect patient outcomes. They recommended that T1 be further divided into T1a (intramucosal carcinoma) and T1b (submucosal carcinoma) and that N1 encompass involvement in one or two regional lymph nodes, with N2 defining involvement in three or more regional lymph nodes. In addition, they found that subclassification of M1 was not useful for predicting prognosis.

Wijnihoven and colleagues[17] published an evaluation of a group of 292 patients who underwent esophagectomy in 2007. In this study, the TNM modifications as proposed by Rice in 2003 more accurately predicted patient survival than the International Union Against Cancer TNM classification. Wijnihoven and colleagues also found that the subclassification of M1 into M1a and M1b was not useful for prognosis in their patient cohort. Thompson and colleagues[18] studied 240 patients who underwent resection for esophageal carcinoma. In this study, the addition of a histologic grade and a change in the "pN" portion of the staging system were identified as changes that could improve the prognostic ability of the TNM system.

CHANGES ASSOCIATED WITH BARRETT ESOPHAGUS: PAGET CELLS ASSOCIATED WITH BARRETT ESOPHAGUS OR WITH ADENOCARCINOMA OF THE ESOPHAGOGASTRIC JUNCTION

Paget disease has been described in several locations, including skin of the breast, vulva, perianal region, and axilla. Abraham and colleagues[19] describe Paget cells in squamous esophageal mucosa overlying areas of Barrett esophagus–associated adenocarcinomas in eight patients. The cases with esophageal Paget cells all showed a poorly differentiated tumor component with dyscohesive cell architecture. Interest-ingly, Abraham and colleagues[19] note that the Pagetoid component of most of the cases in their study were identified only on retrospective case review. A prevalence of 4.9% was calculated based on their study material, which included 103 esophageal adenocarcinomas without Paget cells. Anecdotally, we too have only observed this phenomenon in the esophagus in association with invasive carcinoma, as described by Abraham and colleagues (**Fig. 4**),[20] in contrast to this appearance in the breast

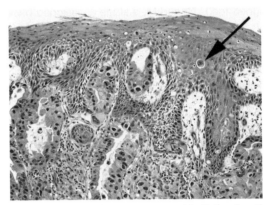

Fig. 4. Carcinoma of the esophagus with squamous reepithelialization. Paget-type cells, such as these (*arrow*) can be identified. The cells represent superficial spread of the underlying invasive carcinoma.

or perineum, where the lesion can truly be an early lesion akin to a skin appendage neoplasm.

ABLATIVE THERAPIES
Photodynamic Therapy

Photodynamic therapy exploits the combined effects of a photosensitizing chemical and specific wavelengths of laser light to produce reactive oxygen species that preferentially ablate tumor tissue by oxidative cellular damage. The targeted tissue is destroyed and reepithelializes with squamous mucosa. The location specificity comes from the uptake of the photosensitizer drug, which preferentially accumulates in tumor tissue.[21] Photosensitizers used today in the treatment of Barrett esophagus–associated dysplasia and carcinoma include hematoporphyrin derivatives and porfimer sodium. These agents are administered intravenously approximately 48 hours before the photoradiation step. Photoradiation itself is performed endoscopically using lasers in conjunction with cylindrical diffusing fibers or localizing balloons. The wavelength of light used depends on the molar absorption coefficient of the photosensitizer compound. The ideal sensitizer compound would only be taken up by the tumor tissue. However, the current photosensitizers are also taken up to varying degrees by other tissues, necessitating that the patients avoid sunlight and excessive room light for weeks after treatment. Despite some such drawbacks, many studies have found that photodynamic therapy compares favorably to esophagectomy as far as overall long-term survival.[22] Because esophagectomy is associated with high morbidity and mortality, this endoscopic alternative is extremely attractive to physicians and patients, and most observers no longer suggest esophagectomy for patients with high-grade dysplasia.[2] Prasad and colleagues[23] studied multiple biomarkers by fluorescence in situ hybridization in 31 patients who underwent photodynamic therapy. They found that after photodynamic therapy there was an association between loss of neoplasia-associated biomarkers (9p21, 17p13.1, 8q24 gains, and others) and histologic downgrading of dysplasia. Patients who did not show loss of biomarkers may be at an increased risk for disease progression. In the future, the pathologist may be able to assist in the direction of treatment and prediction of treatment response based on biomarker results similar to these.

Argon Plasma Coagulation

Argon plasma coagulation, performed endoscopically, makes use of a probe that sends energy through an ionized plasma of argon gas to the tissue without contact with the tissue itself. The energy delivered to the tissue causes ablative damage, termed *coagulation*. The depth of this coagulation is limited to approximately 3 mm.[24,25] The targeted tissue is destroyed and reepithelializes with squamous mucosa. This plasma coagulation method, often used in conjuction with proton pump inhibitor pharmacologic treatment, has been used successfully in the treatment of non-neoplastic Barrett esophagus, but the usefulness of ablation of non-neoplastic Barrett is not well understood.[24,26] Van Laethem and colleagues[25] showed that, when argon plasma coagulation was used for the treatment of Barrett-associated high-grade dysplasia and adenocarcinoma, these lesions were eradicated in 8 of 10 patients.

Multipolar Electrocoagulation

Multipolar electrocoagulation is another endoscopically performed ablative procedure. Like argon plasma coagulation, there is no need for the administration of a sensitizer drug. Multipolar electrocoagulation uses a probe to deliver electrical energy to the tissue via the completion of an electrical circuit between electrodes located at the tip of the probe. The targeted tissue is destroyed and reepithelializes with squamous mucosa. In 2005, Dulai and colleagues[27] reported no statistically significant differences in ablation of Barrett esophagus in patients randomized to receive pantoprazole and multipolar electrocoagulation versus pantoprazole and argon plasma coagulation.

CHANGES ASSOCIATED WITH ABLATIVE THERAPY: HISTOLOGY

The end result of successful ablative therapy is complete eradication of the carcinomatous, dysplastic, or sometimes even the metaplastic (Barrett esophagus) tissue. Evaluation of the postablation esophagus begins at endoscopy, with the examining endoscopist obtaining an in vivo image of the tissue. Histologic evaluation of the post-ablation esophagus is done the same way as an evaluation of an untreated esophagus. Unfortunately, the pathologist is often unaware of the treatment history of the patient at the time of histologic evaluation. There are changes, however, that are characteristic of the postablation esophageal mucosa that require careful histologic evaluation. One such change is the presence of specialized intestinal metaplasia (Barrett esophagus) present deep to the reepithelialized squamous layer (**Fig. 5**). This "buried Barrett" is also referred to as a "pseudoregression" pattern, and is particularly vexing because it is not usually visually evident to the endoscopist during surveillance procedures, underscoring the need for histologic evaluation of biopsies during surveillance. This pseudoregression pattern has also been noted to develop as a response to proton pump inhibitor therapy.[28,29] To examine the neoplastic potential of buried Barrett esophagus, Hornick and colleagues[29] evaluated proliferation rates and DNA characteristics of nonburied Barrett esophagus before photodynamic therapy, nonburied Barrett esophagus after photodynamic therapy, and buried Barrett esophagus after photodynamic therapy in 12 patients. They found that buried Barrett esophagus after photodynamic therapy showed decreased crypt proliferation as compared with non-buried Barrett esophagus and that buried Barrett esophagus following photodynamic therapy shows normal DNA content (even though it often shows abnormalities before photodynamic therapy). This leads to the conclusion that photodynamic therapy may preferentially destroy cells in Barrett esophagus that have DNA abnormalities prone to entry into the dysplasia/carcinoma sequence.[29]

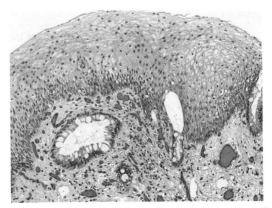

Fig. 5. An area of Barrett esophagus without dysplasia present underneath squamous mucosa, also called buried Barrett or pseudoregression pattern.

Occasionally, buried neoplasia can also be identified (**Fig. 6**), although usually patients with this finding also have some surface neoplasia as well.

CHANGES ASSOCIATED WITH CHEMOTHERAPY AND RADIATION

Chemotherapy and radiation cause characteristic changes in many types of cells, findings that have been observed for years.[30] Characteristic radiation changes include cytoplasmic vacuolization, collagen homogenization, stromal fibroblasts with atypical shapes and sizes, atypical-appearing endothelial cells, small vessel telangiectasia, intimal vascular proliferation, epithelial atrophy, and bizarre nuclear shapes and sizes. Unfortunately, none of these changes are pathognomonic for radiation effect, and each can be caused by multiple types of injury or neoplastic processes. Homogenization of collagen (scarring) can be seen in the lamina propria and submucosal tissue. Atypical fibroblasts, some with bizarre star-shaped nuclei, may appear to be part of a neoplastic process at first glance (**Fig. 7**). In esophageal radiation fields, new

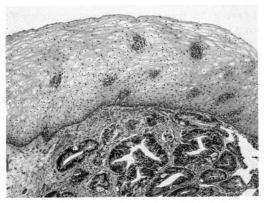

Fig. 6. In this field, the "buried" Barrett esophagus has proceeded to neoplasia. These lesions may be difficult for the endoscopist to detect because the neoplastic cells are hidden beneath a layer of squamous epithelium.

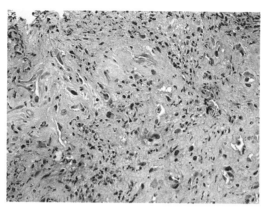

Fig. 7. Atypical stromal cells adjacent to an area of esophageal ulceration after radiation therapy. These enlarged cells are benign. The collagen is dense and homogenized, and some cells are hyperchromatic, with anisocytosis. In some cases, radiation atypia can be mistaken for a neoplastic process.

proliferating vessels tend to orient themselves parallel (rather than perpendicular) to the basement membrane or lumen.

Histologic changes caused by chemotherapy overlap with those associated with radiation treatment and are nonspecific as to agent[31] with one interesting exception. Paclitaxel (Taxol) produces characteristic changes in gastrointestinal tract mucosa that can both be recognized histologically and can be a source of diagnostic errors for pathologists.[32] Paclitaxel induces these gastrointestinal mucosal changes by binding to microtubules, thus promoting polymerization and inhibiting depolymerization. Electron microscopy has shown this central core of polymerized microtubules surrounded by dispersed chromatin, resulting in a "ring" structure during metaphase.[33] The effect can be encountered in patients who have paclitaxel toxicity and in patients who have been administered the medication within about 2 to 4 days. Paclitaxel-associated changes seen on routine histology include numerous ring-shaped (arrested) mitotic figures restricted to the proliferative compartment of the mucosa (**Fig. 8**). In squamous mucosa, this is the basal layer, whereas in columnar mucosa, it is in the area between the base and surface of the mucosa. Mitotic arrest is accompanied by prominent apoptosis. This change is absent at the surface, a clue that the change is not an indication of dysplasia, with which paclitaxel-associated changes are frequently confused.

CHANGES ASSOCIATED WITH CHEMOTHERAPY AND RADIATION: MUCIN POOLS

Some patients who undergo esophagectomy (approximately 10.9%) after chemotherapy and radiation show a puzzling finding: pools of acellular mucin in the esophageal wall.[34] Sometimes these mucin pools contain neoplastic cells. In other cases, the mucin itself is the only vestige of the neoplastic process seen in the specimen. Many of the patients who exhibit this finding had one of two tumor patterns before treatment: mucinous or signet ring.[34] In their 2006 study, Hornick and colleagues[34] showed that the presence of mucin pools alone in these previously treated patients should not be considered residual tumor, even when the mucin pools are located at a resection margin, and that such zones should be staged as pT0 (**Fig. 9**). This was similar to findings reported by Chieieac and colleagues:[35,36] Patients with residual

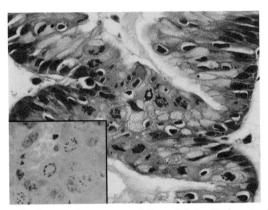

Fig. 8. Paclitaxel (Taxol) changes in an area of Barrett intestinal metaplasia and adjacent squamous esophageal mucosa (*inset*). Numerous ring-shaped (arrested) mitotic figures are seen, accompanied by prominent apoptosis. The changes are restricted to the proliferative compartment, a clue in separating the epithelial changes from dysplasia.

acellular mucin pools on esophagectomy samples taken after chemoradiation were alive at 36 months. Additionally, if signet cell or mucinous histology was found in patients treated by chemoradiation, those patients had a better outcome than that of patients with signet cell or mucinous histology treated by surgery alone.[36] Unfortunately, [(18)F]-fluorodeoxyglucose-positron emission tomography (FDG-PET) imaging is not useful for predicting tumor response.[37]

The utility of using keratin stains to enhance detection of residual carcinoma cells in otherwise acellular mucin pools has not been explored well, although it is not typically difficult to detect epithelial cells in mucin pools by routine (hematoxylin and eosin) histology. Meanwhile, the results of reported studies are inconsistent about the utility of assessing regional lymph nodes with keratin labeling in regional lymph nodes from esophagectomy samples to predict outcome.[38,39] We have not adopted this practice as a reflex test at our institution.

As our colleagues who perform endoscopy refine their sampling techniques with novel real-time methods, such as confocal laser endomicroscopy[40] and other

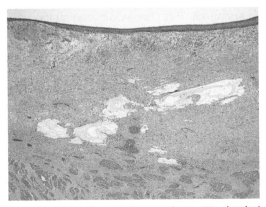

Fig. 9. Mucin pools seen in an esophagectomy specimen. No dysplasia or neoplasia was present in this specimen. The presence of mucin pools alone does not constitute residual tumor, even when present at resection margins.

modalities, and as we learn to screen for and better detect early lesions, we expect that pathologists and gastroenterologists alike will refine staging of early lesions and gather better prognostic information to allow us to improve care of our patients.

REFERENCES

1. Jemal A, Siegel R, Ward E, et al. Cancer statistics, 2008. CA Cancer J Clin 2008; 58(2):71–96.
2. Wang KK, Sampliner RE. Updated guidelines 2008 for the diagnosis, surveillance and therapy of Barrett's esophagus. Am J Gastroenterol 2008;103(3):788–97.
3. Rubio CA, Riddell R. Musculo-fibrous anomaly in Barrett's mucosa with dysplasia. Am J Surg Pathol 1988;12(11):885–9.
4. Rubio CA, Aberg B. Further studies on the musculo-fibrous anomaly of the Barrett's mucosa in esophageal carcinomas. Pathol Res Pract 1991;187(8):1009–13.
5. Tada T, Suzuki T, Iwafuchi M, et al. Adenocarcinoma arising in Barrett's esophagus after total gastrectomy. Am J Gastroenterol 1990;85(11):1503–6.
6. Nishimaki T, Holscher AH, Schuler M, et al. Chronic esophagitis and subsequent morphological changes of the esophageal mucosa in Barrett's esophagus: a histological study of esophagectomy specimens. Surg Today 1994;24(3):203–9.
7. Takubo K, Sasajima K, Yamashita K, et al. Double muscularis mucosae in Barrett's esophagus. Hum Pathol 1991;22(11):1158–61.
8. Hahn HP, Shahsafaei A, Odze RD. Vascular and lymphatic properties of the superficial and deep lamina propria in Barrett esophagus. Am J Surg Pathol 2008;32(10):1454–61.
9. Westerterp M, Koppert LB, Buskens CJ, et al. Outcome of surgical treatment for early adenocarcinoma of the esophagus or gastro-esophageal junction. Virchows Arch 2005;446(5):497–504.
10. Abraham SC, Krasinskas AM, Correa AM, et al. Duplication of the muscularis mucosae in Barrett esophagus: an underrecognized feature and its implication for staging of adenocarcinoma. Am J Surg Pathol 2007;31(11):1719–25.
11. Larghi A, Lightdale CJ, Memeo L, et al. EUS followed by EMR for staging of high-grade dysplasia and early cancer in Barrett's esophagus. Gastrointest Endosc 2005;62(1):16–23.
12. Liu L, Hofstetter WL, Rashid A, et al. Significance of the depth of tumor invasion and lymph node metastasis in superficially invasive (T1) esophageal adenocarcinoma. Am J Surg Pathol 2005;29(8):1079–85.
13. Japanese Society for Esophageal Diseases. Guidelines for clinical and pathologic studies. Carcinoma of the esophagus. 9th edition. Tokyo: Kanehara; 2001.
14. Joint Committee on Cancer A. AJCC cancer staging handbook. 6th edition. Philadelphia: Lippincott-Raven; 2002.
15. Sobin LH. TNM: evolution and relation to other prognostic factors. Semin Surg Oncol 2003;21(1):3–7.
16. Rice TW, Blackstone EH, Rybicki LA, et al. Refining esophageal cancer staging. J Thorac Cardiovasc Surg 2003;125(5):1103–13.
17. Wijnhoven BP, Tran KT, Esterman A, et al. An evaluation of prognostic factors and tumor staging of resected carcinoma of the esophagus. Ann Surg 2007;245(5):717–25.
18. Thompson SK, Ruszkiewicz AR, Jamieson GG, et al. Improving the accuracy of TNM staging in esophageal cancer: a pathological review of resected specimens. Ann Surg Oncol 2008;15:3447–58.

19. Abraham SC, Wang H, Wang KK, et al. Paget cells in the esophagus: assessment of their histopathologic features and near-universal association with underlying esophageal adenocarcinoma. Am J Surg Pathol 2008;32(7):1068–74.

20. Goldblum JR, Hart WR. Perianal Paget's disease: a histologic and immunohisto-chemical study of 11 cases with and without associated rectal adenocarcinoma. Am J Surg Pathol 1998;22(2):170–9.

21. Dolmans DE, Fukumura D, Jain RK. Photodynamic therapy for cancer. Nat Rev Cancer 2003;3(5):380–7.

22. Prasad GA, Wang KK, Buttar NS, et al. Long-term survival following endoscopic and surgical treatment of high-grade dysplasia in Barrett's esophagus. Gastroen-terology 2007;132(4):1226–33.

23. Prasad GA, Wang KK, Halling KC, et al. Correlation of histology with biomarker status after photodynamic therapy in Barrett esophagus. Cancer 2008;113(3):470–6.

24. Franchimont D, Van Laethem JL, Deviere J. Argon plasma coagulation in Barrett's esophagus. Gastrointest Endosc Clin N Am 2003;13(3):457–66.

25. Van Laethem JL, Jagodzinski R, Peny MO, et al. Argon plasma coagulation in the treatment of Barrett's high-grade dysplasia and in situ adenocarcinoma. Endos-copy 2001;33(3):257–61.

26. Manner H, May A, Miehlke S, et al. Ablation of nonneoplastic Barrett's mucosa using argon plasma coagulation with concomitant esomeprazole therapy (APBANEX): a prospective multicenter evaluation. Am J Gastroenterol 2006; 101(8):1762–9.

27. Dulai GS, Jensen DM, Cortina G, et al. Randomized trial of argon plasma coag-ulation vs. multipolar electrocoagulation for ablation of Barrett's esophagus. Gas-trointest Endosc 2005;61(2):232–40.

28. Hornick JL, Blount PL, Sanchez CA, et al. Biologic properties of columnar epithe-lium underneath reepithelialized squamous mucosa in Barrett's esophagus. Am J Surg Pathol 2005;29(3):372–80.

29. Hornick JL, Mino-Kenudson M, Lauwers GY, et al. Buried Barrett's epithelium following photodynamic therapy shows reduced crypt proliferation and absence of DNA content abnormalities. Am J Gastroenterol 2008;103(1):38–47.

30. Berthrong M, Fajardo LF. Radiation injury in surgical pathology. Part II. Alimentary tract. Am J Surg Pathol 1981;5(2):153–78.

31. O'Morchoe PJ, Lee DC, Kozak CA. Esophageal cytology in patients receiving cytotoxic drug therapy. Acta Cytol 1983;27(6):630–4.

32. Daniels JA, Gibson MK, Xu L, et al. Gastrointestinal tract epithelial changes asso-ciated with taxanes: marker of drug toxicity versus effect. Am J Surg Pathol 2008; 32(3):473–7.

33. Hruban RH, Yardley JH, Donehower RC, et al. Taxol toxicity. Epithelial necrosis in the gastrointestinal tract associated with polymerized microtubule accumulation and mitotic arrest. Cancer 1989;63(10):1944–50.

34. Hornick JL, Farraye FA, Odze RD. Prevalence and significance of prominent mucin pools in the esophagus post neoadjuvant chemoradiotherapy for Bar-rett's-associated adenocarcinoma. Am J Surg Pathol 2006;30(1):28–35.

35. Chirieac LR, Swisher SG, Ajani JA, et al. Posttherapy pathologic stage predicts survival in patients with esophageal carcinoma receiving preoperative chemora-diation. Cancer 2005;103(7):1347–55.

36. Chirieac LR, Swisher SG, Correa AM, et al. Signet-ring cell or mucinous histology after preoperative chemoradiation and survival in patients with esophageal or esophagogastric junction adenocarcinoma. Clin Cancer Res 2005;11(6): 2229–36.

37. Gillham CM, Lucey JA, Keogan M, et al. (18)FDG uptake during induction chemo-radiation for oesophageal cancer fails to predict histomorphological tumour response. Br J Cancer 2006;95(9):1174–9.
38. Heeren PA, Kelder W, Blondeel I, et al. Prognostic value of nodal micrometasta-ses in patients with cancer of the gastro-oesophageal junction. Eur J Surg Oncol 2005;31(3):270–6.
39. Waterman TA, Hagen JA, Peters JH, et al. The prognostic importance of immuno-histochemically detected node metastases in resected esophageal adenocarci-noma. Ann Thorac Surg 2004;78(4):1161–9 [discussion: 1161–9].
40. Kiesslich R, Gossner L, Goetz M, et al. In vivo histology of Barrett's esophagus and associated neoplasia by confocal laser endomicroscopy. Clin Gastroenterol Hepatol 2006;4(8):979–87.

Preoperative Therapy for Esophageal Cancer

Geoffrey Y. Ku, MD[a], David H. Ilson, MD, PhD[b,*]

KEYWORDS

- Esophageal cancer • Preoperative therapy • Chemotherapy
- Chemoradiotherapy • PET scan

In the United States, esophageal cancer is an uncommon but aggressive malignancy. In 2008, an estimated 16,470 patients were diagnosed, with an estimated 14,280 deaths from this disease. It is the seventh leading cause of cancer death in men.[1] Globally, both esophageal and gastric cancers account for an estimated 1.4 million new cases and 1.1 million cancer deaths, more than colorectal and breast cancer combined.[2]

Squamous cell carcinoma (SCC) and adenocarcinoma account for 98% of all cases of esophageal cancer. Although cases of SCC have declined steadily, the incidence of adenocarcinoma of the distal esophagus, gastroesophageal (GE) junction, and gastric cardia has increased 4% to 10% per year among men in the United States since 1976 so that it is now the most common histology.[3,4] Currently, both the SCC and adenocarcinoma histologies are treated similarly, although there are increasing data that both histologies respond differently to chemotherapy and chemoradiotherapy respectively.

For locally advanced esophageal cancer, surgery remains the mainstay of treatment. Various reviews have reported 5-year overall survival (OS) rates from 10% up to 30% to 40% with surgical resection alone.[5,6] Primary radiation therapy previously was used for local tumor control, although less successfully. In one large series, the 3-year survival after radiotherapy alone was only 6%.[7] For metastatic disease, chemotherapy alone results in response rates of only 20% to 40% and median survivals of 8 to 10 months.[8]

Given the activity of all three modalities, numerous studies have combined them in distinct neoadjuvant (preoperative) strategies for locally advanced disease. Multimodality approaches have included chemotherapy or concurrent chemoradiotherapy followed by surgery or definitive chemoradiotherapy, in an effort to improve the dismal prognosis of this aggressive cancer. Relatively few studies have focused on an adjuvant (postoperative) approach.

[a] Ludwig Center for Cancer Immunotherapy, Memorial Sloan-Kettering Cancer Center, 1275 York Avenue, New York, NY 10065, USA
[b] Gastrointestinal Oncology Service, Department of Medicine, Memorial Sloan-Kettering Cancer Center, 1275 York Avenue, New York, NY 10065, USA
* Corresponding author.
E-mail address: ilsond@mskcc.org (D.H. Ilson).

Gastroenterol Clin N Am 38 (2009) 135–152
doi:10.1016/j.gtc.2009.01.012
0889-8553/09/$ – see front matter © 2009 Elsevier Inc. All rights reserved.

The results of these studies have been mixed, and their combined outcomes have failed to elevate any preoperative strategies to a clear standard for resectable esophageal cancer. Recent trials involving preoperative chemoradiotherapy and pre- and peri-operative chemotherapy, however, have demonstrated improved survival over surgery alone. Based on these data, many clinicians now treat locoregional disease with preoperative multimodality therapy.

NEOADJUVANT CHEMOTHERAPY

Despite the short-lived responses using chemotherapy alone in advanced disease, neoadjuvant chemotherapy is associated with many theoretical benefits.[9] This approach has the potential to assess tumor response to chemotherapy and direct the possible use of chemotherapy postoperatively. Chemotherapy also may improve baseline dysphagia, downstage the primary tumor, and increase resection rates and treat micrometastatic disease that is undetectable at diagnosis.

Kok and colleagues[10] reported a small randomized phase three trial, in which 148 patients who had SCC were randomized to surgery alone or preoperative cisplatin/etoposide followed by surgery. Preoperative chemotherapy was associated with a significant improvement in median OS (18.5 months versus 11 months). No final report of this study has been published.

The large North American Intergroup 113 trial, however, failed to show a survival benefit for peri-operative cisplatin/5-fluorouracil (5-FU) plus surgery compared with surgery alone in 440 patients who had adenocarcinoma and squamous cell carcinoma.[11] Patients in the combined-modality arm received three cycles of cisplatin/5-FU preoperatively and two cycles postoperatively. Pathologic complete responses (pCR) were seen in only 2.5% of patients receiving preoperative chemotherapy, and there was no improvement in the curative resection rate. The median OS was not significantly different in the two groups, and the 5-year OS with or without chemotherapy was 20%. The addition of chemotherapy did not change the rate of recurrence either locally or at distant sites. Outcome also did not differ by histology, with no benefit seen for preoperative chemotherapy for either adenocarcinoma or SCC.

Renewed interest in preoperative chemotherapy was generated by a trial performed by the Medical Research Council Esophageal Cancer Working Group.[12] This study randomized 802 patients (nearly double the number of patients in the Intergroup trial) to surgery alone versus two cycles of preoperative cisplatin/5-FU. At a relatively short median follow-up of only 2 years, the chemotherapy-treated group demonstrated improved median OS (16.8 months versus 13.3 months) and 2-year survival (43% versus 34%). The curative resection rate was improved marginally from 55% to 60%, and the pCR rate was 4% in the preoperative therapy group. Mature results of this trial recently were updated in abstract form.[13] At 5 years, there continued to be a statistically significant but numerically smaller OS benefit for preoperative therapy (23% versus 17%). The trial reported a sobering operative mortality rate of 10%.

It may be that the larger sample size compared with the Intergroup trial facilitated the detection of a small improvement with chemotherapy. In addition, a larger proportion of patients on this trial had adenocarcinoma histology compared with the Intergroup 113 trial (66% versus 54%). Two recent meta-analyses (described in detail) suggest a potentially greater survival benefit from preoperative chemotherapy for patients who have adenocarcinoma versus SCC.[14,15]

Additional evidence to support the use of peri-operative chemotherapy comes from the recent Medical Research Council Adjuvant Gastric Infusional Chemotherapy (MAGIC) trial performed in the United Kingdom.[16] This trial randomized 503 patients who had gastric or gastroesophageal (GE) junction adenocarcinoma to three cycles each of pre- and postoperative ECF (epirubicin/cisplatin/infusional 5-FU) chemo-therapy and surgery or surgery alone. peri-operative chemotherapy resulted in significant improvement in 5-year OS (36% versus 23%). There was no improvement, however, in the curative resection rate, and there were no cases of pCR. Although only 26% of patients on this trial had tumors in the GE junction and lower esophagus, the results still may apply to esophageal cancer.

Finally, data from the French FFCD 9703 trial of 224 patients who had gastric or lower esophageal adenocarcinoma recently were presented.[17] Patients were randomized to two or three cycles of preoperative cisplatin/5-FU followed by surgery versus surgery alone. Those patients who appeared to benefit clinically or radiographically from preoperative therapy or who had persistent T3 or node-positive disease at surgery also received an additional three or four cycles of chemotherapy. Preoperative chemotherapy was associated with a significant improvement in R0 resection rate (84% versus 73%), 5-year disease-free survival (DFS, 34% versus 21%) and 5-year OS (38% versus 24%). Although comparisons between different clinical trials must be made cautiously, the survival benefit seen with preoperative cisplatin/5-FU on this trial appears to be very similar to that seen with peri-operative ECF in the MAGIC trial. Because of the smaller sample size on this trial, however, outcome differences in as few as 10 to 15 patients would have changed the trial outcome. Also, the trial did not stage patients with endoscopic ultrasound consistently or stratify them by pretherapy stage. In a small-scale trial, even a slight imbalance in pretherapy stage might impact the trial outcome.

These data are summarized in **Table 1**. Overall, recent trials suggest a survival benefit for peri-operative chemotherapy, although preoperative chemotherapy alone is associated with a low pCR rate and inconsistent improvement in the resection rate. Such a survival benefit also was demonstrated in a recent large, individual patient data meta-analysis of 12 randomized trials involving preoperative chemotherapy.[15] This meta-analysis revealed a 5-year survival benefit of only 4% with preoperative chemotherapy, with a suggestion of lesser benefit for squamous (4%) compared with adenocarcinoma histology (7%).

Neoadjuvant Radiation Therapy

Trials that have evaluated the use of preoperative radiation have largely reported no benefit.

Kelsen and colleagues[18] performed a randomized trial comparing preoperative radiation to preoperative chemotherapy in 96 patients with esophageal cancer. Although there was no increase in operative morbidity or mortality for patients treated with preoperative therapy compared with historical controls treated with surgery alone, there was also no additional treatment benefit. Another randomized trial involving 176 patients also failed to identify a benefit for preoperative radiation.[19]

A prospective, multicenter Scandinavian trial reported by Nygaard and colleagues[20] randomized 186 patients who had esophageal SCC to four treatment groups: surgery alone, preoperative chemotherapy (cisplatin/bleomycin) and surgery, preoperative radiation and surgery, or preoperative chemotherapy and radiation, followed by surgery. The 3-year OS was significantly higher in the pooled groups receiving radiation compared with the nonradiation groups. The results indicated an intermediate-term survival benefit for preoperative radiation but found that chemotherapy did not influence survival.

A subsequent meta-analysis, however, was unable to establish a significant benefit for preoperative radiation.[21] With a median follow-up of 9 years, an analysis of more

Table 1
Results of phase 3 preoperative chemotherapy trials in esophageal cancer

Treatment	Histology	Number of Patients	R0 Resection Rate	Pathologic Complete Response Rate	Survival		Local Failure	Reference
					Median	Overall		
Surgery	SCC	41	37%	N/A	NS	3 y 9%	NS	Nygaard et al[20]
Cis/bleo + surgery		50	44%	NS		3 y 3%		
RT + surgery		48	55%			3 y 21%		
Cis/bleo/RT + surgery		47	44%			3 y 17%		
Cis/etop+ surgery	SCC	74	NS	NS	18.5 months	NS	NS	Kok et al[10]
Surgery		74		N/A	11 months			
Peri-operative Cis/5FU + surgery	SCC (46%) + adeno (54%)	213	62%	2.5%	14.9 months	3 y 23%	32%	Kelsen et al[11]
Surgery		227	59%	N/A	16.1 months	3 y 26%	31%	
Preoperative Cis/5FU + surgery	SCC (31%) + adeno (66%)	400	60%	NS	16.8 months	2 y 43% 5 y 23%	13%	Medical Research Council[12,13]
Surgery		402	54%	N/A	13.3 months	2 y 34% 5 y 17%	11%	
Peri-operative ECF + surgery	Adeno	250	69%	0%	24 months	5 y 36%	14%	Cunningham et al[16]
Surgery		253	66%	N/A	20 months	5 y 23%	21%	
Peri-operative Cis/5FU + surgery	Adeno	113	87%	3%	NS	5 y 38%	NS	Boige et al[17]
Surgery		111	74%	N/A	NS	5 y 24%	NS	

Abbreviations: Adeno, adenocarcinoma; bleo, bleomycin; cis, cisplatin; ECF, epirubicin, cisplatin, 5-fluorouracil; etop, etoposide; 5FU, 5-fluorouracil; N/A, not applicable; NS, not stated; RT, radiotherapy; SCC, squamous cell carcinoma.

than 1100 patients from five randomized trials suggested a survival benefit of 3% at 2 years and 4% at 5 years that was not statistically significant ($P = .062$).

Adjuvant Therapy

Combined-modality therapy in esophageal carcinoma long has focused on preoperative strategies. The role of adjuvant therapy has not been studied extensively, and the data that are available suggest equivocal results.

Postoperative chemotherapy without preoperative therapy was studied in two Japanese randomized trials, where patients who had SCC histology were randomized to receive two cycles of chemotherapy with cisplatin/vindesine[22] or cisplatin/5-FU[23] respectively. Although the trial with cisplatin/vindesine did not show any survival benefit, an unplanned subset analysis of the trial with cisplatin/5-FU revealed a survival benefit for patients who had lymph node involvement (5-year DFS 52% versus 38%).

The possible benefit for postoperative therapy suggested by the previously mentioned trials led to a subsequent Japanese trial that randomized 330 patients who had SCC histology to surgery and either two cycles of pre- or postoperative cisplatin/5-FU.[24] Data recently presented in abstract form revealed that preoperative chemotherapy was associated with a significant improvement in OS compared with postoperative chemotherapy (hazard ratio [HR] 0.64, 95% CI, 0.45 to 0.91), further questioning the role of adjuvant chemotherapy for SCC. A significant number of patients on this trial, however, never received postoperative chemotherapy, making the results difficult to interpret. Another unexpected finding is that an unplanned subset analysis suggested that the benefit for preoperative therapy over postoperative therapy was seen only in patients without lymph node involvement, in contrast to the previously mentioned study where a benefit for adjuvant chemotherapy over observation was noted in patients who had lymph node involvement.

The overall lack of benefit for adjuvant chemotherapy suggested by the Japanese trials is consistent with the results of a randomized French trial, which also found no survival benefit for 6 to 8 months of adjuvant chemotherapy with cisplatin/5-FU.[25] In fact, there were significantly more complications in the chemotherapy group.

In contrast, a pilot Eastern Cooperative Oncology Group (ECOG) trial recently evaluated four cycles of postoperative paclitaxel/cisplatin in patients who had node-positive esophageal or GE junction adenocarcinoma.[26] Two-year OS was 60%, which is statistically superior compared with the historical control (38%, derived from Intergroup 113 trial).

Trials involving adjuvant radiotherapy generally have reported negative results. A French study randomized 221 patients to surgery alone versus surgery followed by radiation and found no survival benefit from radiation.[27]

Another randomized study of 130 patients from Hong Kong actually demonstrated increased mortality with postoperative radiation (8.7 versus 15.2 months, in favor of the no adjuvant therapy group), with the difference attributed to radiation-related deaths and early metastatic disease.[28]

Finally, a large prospective Chinese study also failed to detect an OS benefit among 495 patients randomized to adjuvant radiation or no further therapy.[29] A subgroup analysis of node-positive patients, however, did show a 5-year OS benefit favoring the radiation group (35.1% versus 13.1%).

Although trials of adjuvant radiotherapy alone have not suggested significant benefit, there may be benefit from adjuvant concurrent chemoradiotherapy, as suggested the results of the Intergroup trial 116 in gastric adenocarcinoma.[30] This trial revealed a significant improvement in OS and DFS for the delivery of postoperative therapy with 5-FU/leucovorin and radiation compared with surgery alone. As a relatively modest 20% of the patients treated had proximal gastric cancers (with involvement of the GE junction) and primary GE junction cancers, these data may justify the use of postoperative therapy in such patients who have not received preoperative therapy. It should be noted that the results of this trial have been questioned because of the relatively inadequate surgical resections that were performed; 54% of patients had a D0 resection, which is less than a complete dissection of the involved lymph nodes. It has been argued that radiation in this setting compensated for inadequate surgery and that its benefits may not be seen if a more complete or extensive D1 or D2 surgical resection is undertaken.

Combined Neoadjuvant Chemoradiotherapy

Although recent pre- and peri-operative chemotherapy trials have indicated a survival benefit, the low rate of pCR and the inconsistent impact on rates of operability have led researchers to investigate neoadjuvant chemoradiotherapy.

Chemoradiotherapy typically involves regimens of cisplatin or mitomycin and continuous infusion 5-FU, with radiotherapy dosages from 30 to 40 Gy and up to 60 Gy in more recent trials. Such therapy results in pCR rates of 20% to 40%, with long-term survival of no more than 25% to 35%.[31,32] Superior survival is achieved consistently, though in patients achieving a pCR to chemoradiotherapy (up to 50% to 60% at 5 years).[33–37]

These results are at the expense of significant toxicities, primarily hematologic and gastrointestinal (GI), which have been greatest in trials employing a higher dose of or twice-daily radiation or in which radiotherapy overlapped all cycles of preoperative chemotherapy.[38] The GI toxicity associated with cisplatin/5-FU and radiation includes nausea, mucositis, and esophagitis, leading some investigators to mandate placement of enteral feeding tubes before treatment initiation.

The seminal phase 3 United States Radiation Therapy Oncology Group (RTOG) trial 85-01 demonstrated the superiority of chemoradiotherapy over radiation alone.[39] This nonoperative study compared standard-fractionation radiation (64 Gy) with radiation (50 Gy) plus concurrent cisplatin/5-FU. The trial was stopped when data from 121 patients showed an improved median OS in favor of chemoradiotherapy (12.5 months versus 8.9 months). Two-year survival was also improved in the chemoradiotherapy group (38% versus 10%), as was 5-year survival (21% versus 0%).[40] Although most patents treated on this trial had SCC, long-term survival also was seen in the small number of adenocarcinoma patients on the trial, with 13% of patients alive at 5 years.

In addition to a survival benefit, disease recurrence was reduced significantly by the addition of chemotherapy to radiation. At 1 year, recurrent disease was observed in 62% of the group that received radiation versus 44% in the chemoradiotherapy arm. Distant recurrence rates were 38% and 22%, respectively. Based on this study, chemoradiotherapy was established as the standard of care in the nonsurgical management of locally advanced esophageal SCC.

Building on these results, more intensive treatment strategies have been investigated. In the nonoperative RTOG 90-12 chemoradiotherapy study, induction chemotherapy with cisplatin/5-FU followed by chemoradiotherapy with the same regimen did not appear to afford any additional benefit.[41] The RTOG 94-05 study compared a total radiation dose of 64.8 Gy versus 50.4 Gy during concurrent cisplatin/5-FU and also failed to demonstrate superior results with the more intense regimen.[42] This study confirmed 50.4 Gy as the standard radiation dose when given in combined therapy with cisplatin/5-FU. Finally, the phase 1/2 RTOG 92-07 trial, which attempted to boost radiation with brachytherapy following external beam radiation, revealed significant toxicity, including a 12% incidence of treatment-related fistulas.[43]

Phase 3 Trials of Chemoradiotherapy

Five contemporary randomized trials have compared preoperative chemoradiotherapy followed by surgery versus surgery alone. The results are summarized in **Table 2**.

Urba and colleagues[44] from the University of Michigan randomized 100 patients to preoperative cisplatin/5-FU/vinblastine and radiation or to surgery alone. Despite a statistically significant decrease in the rate of local recurrence favoring preoperative therapy (19% versus 42%), 3-year OS trended toward improvement but was not statistically significant (30% versus 16%, $P = .15$). Rates of curative resection were equivalent in both groups (90%). Most patients treated on this trial had adenocarcinoma.

Walsh and associates from Ireland randomized 113 patients who had esophageal adenocarcinoma to preoperative cisplatin/5-FU/radiation or surgery alone.[45] Rates of negative margin resection were not reported, although it was noted that the preoperative therapy group had a significantly lower incidence of positive lymph nodes or metastatic disease at surgery (42% versus 82%). A significant improvement in 3-year OS was noted (32% versus 6%). Interpretation of this study is confounded by the very poor survival of the surgical control arm—6% at 3 years—which is inconsistent with the approximate 20% 5-year survival rates reported for modern surgical series.[46] Other shortcomings of this trial include inadequate pretherapy staging that could have led to an imbalance in prognostic factors between both groups, the variable surgical procedures used, premature termination based on an unplanned interim analysis, and the relatively short follow-up period for surviving patients (18 months).

Bosset and colleagues,[47] on behalf of the European Organization for Research and Treatment of Cancer (EORTC), randomized 282 patients with esophageal SCC to preoperative cisplatin and concurrent split-dose radiation or surgery. Compared with the surgery-only group, the chemoradiotherapy group had a significantly higher rate of curative resection (81% versus 69%), and an improvement in disease-free survival and a decreased risk of local recurrence. OS (the primary trial endpoint), however, was not significantly different. It might be that the significantly higher postoperative mortality in the chemoradiotherapy arm (12% versus 4%) outweighed any potential survival benefit for the chemoradiotherapy group.

In an Australian trial, Burmeister and colleagues[48] randomized 256 patients to one cycle of preoperative cisplatin/5-FU and radiation or to surgery alone. Although the trial failed to show a survival advantage for patients who received chemoradiotherapy, they did have a significantly higher curative resection rate compared with the surgery-only patients (80% versus 59%). In this study, the administration of a single chemotherapy cycle may represent suboptimal delivery of chemotherapy, as suggested by the unexpectedly low pCR rate in the adenocarcinoma patients of only 9%.

Finally, results of the Cancer and Leukemia Group B (CALGB) trial 9781 recently were published.[49] This trial randomized patients to two cycles of preoperative cisplatin/5-FU and radiation or to surgery alone. Fifty-six patients were randomized before the trial was closed for poor accrual. Nevertheless, patients assigned to chemoradiotherapy had substantially improved median survival (4.5 versus 1.8 years) and 5-year OS (39% versus 16%) compared with patients undergoing surgery alone.

Overall, these randomized trials are associated with methodological concerns (including the lack of rigorous pretherapy staging with endoscopic ultrasound or laparoscopy), are significantly smaller than randomized preoperative chemotherapy trials, and produce conflicting results. They do suggest improved curative resection rates and decreased local recurrence, however. A survival advantage for preoperative

Table 2
Results of phase 3 preoperative chemoradiotherapy trials in esophageal cancer

Treatment	Histology	Number of Patients	R0 Resection Rate	Pathologic Complete Rate	Survival Median	Overall	Local Failure	Reference
Preoperative CRT	SCC (24%) + adeno (76%)	50	45%	28% (SCC 38%, adeno 24%)	16.9 months	3 y 30%	19%	Urba et al[144]
Surgery		50	45%	N/A	17.6 months	3 y 16%	42%	
Preoperative CRT	Adeno	58	NS	25%	16 months	3 y 32%	NS	Walsh et al[145]
Surgery		55		N/A	11 months	3 y 6%		
Preoperative CRT	SCC	143	81%	26%	18.6 months	5 y 26%	NS	Bosset et al[147]
Surgery		139	69%	N/A	18.6 months	5 y 26%		
Preoperative CRT	SCC (35%) + adeno (63%) + other (2%)	128	80%	16% (SCC 27%, adeno 9%)	22.2 months	NS	15%	Burmeister et al[148]
Surgery		128	59%	N/A	19.3 months	NS	26%	
Preoperative CRT	SCC (25%) + adeno (75%)	30	NS	40%	4.5 years	5 y 39%	NS	Tepper et al[149]
Surgery		26		N/A	1.8 years	5 y 16%	NS	

Abbreviations: Adeno, adenocarcinoma; CRT, chemoradiotherapy; NS, not stated; CRT, SCC, squamous cell carcinoma.

chemoradiotherapy over surgery alone is not demonstrated clearly, although several studies suggest such a trend.

These observations are supported further by a recent meta-analysis, in which 10 randomized trials of preoperative chemoradiotherapy versus surgery alone and eight trials of preoperative chemotherapy versus surgery alone were analyzed.[14] Preoperative chemoradiotherapy was associated with a hazard ratio of all-cause mortality of 0.81 versus surgery alone (95% CI, 0.70 to 0.93, $P = .002$), which translated to a 13% absolute difference in mortality at 2 years. This benefit was irrespective of histology. Preoperative chemotherapy was associated with a hazard ratio of 0.90 (95% CI, 0.81 to 1.00, $P = .05$) compared with surgery alone, which related to a 2-year absolute survival benefit of 7%. There did not appear to be any benefit of preoperative chemotherapy for patients who had squamous histology (hazard ratio 0.88; 95% CI, 0.75 to 1.03, $P = .12$), although there was a benefit for patients who had adenocarcinoma histology (hazard ratio 0.78; 95% CI, 0.64 to 0.95, $P = .014$).

The possible superiority of preoperative chemoradiotherapy over preoperative chemotherapy also has been suggested by a randomized study recently presented in abstract form.[50] In this study by Stahl and colleagues for the German Esophageal Cancer Study Group, patients were randomized to preoperative chemotherapy with cisplatin/5-FU/leucovorin followed by surgery versus cisplatin/5-FU/leucovorin followed by chemoradiotherapy with cisplatin/etoposide and then surgery. One hundred-twenty eligible patients were randomized before the trial was closed because of poor accrual. The results revealed a trend toward improved local progression-free survival (PFS; 77% versus 59%), median OS (32.8 versus 21.1 months), and 3-year survival (43% versus 27%) for the chemoradiotherapy over chemotherapy group, but these results were not statistically significant ($P = .14$). Both the pCR rate (16% versus 2%) and node-negative status (64% versus 37%) were significantly higher in the chemoradiotherapy group. Strengths of this trial include the careful pretherapy staging (which included endoscopic ultrasound and laparoscopy), the enrollment only of high-risk patients with at least T3 or node-positive tumors and the careful balancing of pretherapy stage between the two treatment arms.

Definitive Chemoradiotherapy Versus Chemoradiotherapy Followed by Surgery

Two recent randomized trials have compared definitive chemoradiotherapy versus chemoradiotherapy followed by surgery. The first study was performed by the German Esophageal Cancer Study Group, which assigned 172 patients who had SCC to preoperative therapy (three cycles of cisplatin/5-FU/leucovorin/etoposide, then cisplatin/etoposide and concurrent radiation to 40 Gy) followed by surgery or to the preoperative therapy alone with a higher radiation dose (to at least 65 Gy) in lieu of surgery.[37] Although local PFS was improved with the addition of surgery (HR for chemoradiotherapy-only group versus surgery group 2.1, 95% CI, 1.3 to 3.5, $P = .003$), there was only a nonsignificant trend toward improvement in 3-year OS (31.3% versus 24.4%). Treatment-related mortality was also significantly higher in the surgery group compared with the chemoradiotherapy-only group (12.8% versus 3.5%). Ten-year survival data for this trial recently was presented in abstract form, reaffirming the absence of a significant difference between both groups.[51]

The second study is the French FFCD 9102 trial, where 444 eligible patients who had mostly SCC histology underwent initial chemoradiotherapy with cisplatin/5-FU.[52] Those who responded to initial therapy then were randomized either to undergo surgery or to receive an additional three cycles of cisplatin/5-FU with radiation, as the authors felt that it would be inappropriate to continue chemoradiotherapy in patients not responding to therapy. Of the 444 patients, 259 were randomized.

The 2-year survival rate was not significantly different between both groups (34% in surgery group versus 40% in chemoradiotherapy-only group, $P = .44$). Locoregional recurrence, however, was higher in the chemoradiotherapy-only group (43% versus 34%), and there was also a higher incidence of stent placement in this group (32% versus 5%). Three-month mortality was significantly higher in the surgery group (9.3% versus 0.8%). Based on these data, the authors concluded that patients who have tumors, especially of SCC histology, that respond to initial chemoradiotherapy did not derive any survival benefit from subsequent surgery. Patients who underwent surgery did have improved local control of their disease, albeit at the cost of increased treatment-related mortality.

An interesting question that arises from this study is whether patients who do not respond to initial therapy benefit from subsequent surgery. In a recent abstract, the authors discussed the outcome of the 192 of the 451 registered patients from the previous study who were not randomized to further protocol therapy after initial chemotherapy primarily because of a lack of response but also because of medical contraindication or patient refusal.[53] Of these nonrandomized patients, 112 subsequently underwent surgery, with 80 undergoing R0 resections. The median OS for the patients who underwent surgery was significantly superior to the median OS of those who did not (17.3 versus 6.1 months) and was comparable to the median OS of the patients who were randomized. Although there are clear limitations and potential strong confounders to such an analysis, these data may suggest that salvage esophagectomy can be beneficial for a subset of patients who do not respond to initial therapy.

As a related issue, definitive chemoradiotherapy alone versus surgery alone also recently was compared in a Scandinavian phase 3 trial of 91 patients with adenocarcinoma and SCC who were randomized to receive either cisplatin/5-FU and radiation alone or surgery.[54] At a median follow-up of 51.8 months, there was no survival difference between both groups. Although this study may be underpowered to detect small survival differences, the data collectively support definitive chemoradiotherapy as an acceptable approach for patients who have contraindications to surgery.

NEWER CHEMORADIOTHERAPY REGIMENS

The poor results, and toxicity of therapy, obtained with conventional cisplatin/5-FU-based regimens have led to the search for more effective and better-tolerated regimens.

Paclitaxel-based chemotherapy has undergone extensive evaluation in combined-modality therapy trials with radiation. These phase 2 trials have combined a conventional schedule of paclitaxel/cisplatin every 3 weeks,[55,56] weekly paclitaxel with cisplatin every 3 weeks,[57] or weekly paclitaxel with weekly cisplatin[58,59] or with weekly carboplatin.[60] They have reported pCR rates of 19% to 46%, with toxicities generally less in trials with weekly chemotherapy regimens. Consistently, pCR rates in recent trials are higher in patients who had squamous cancer compared with patients who had adenocarcinoma histology.[48]

Other trials have combined paclitaxel and continuous infusion 5-FU and cisplatin or carboplatin.[61–64] These three-drug trials have reported substantial toxicities, including severe myelosuppression and esophagitis, but they have not consistently demonstrated superior results. Retrospective data from the Massachusetts General Hospital indicated similar pCR rates and 3-year survival for a three-drug regimen of paclitaxel/cisplatin/5-FU and radiation compared with cisplatin/5-FU and radiation.[65]

The relative efficacy and toxicity of paclitaxel-based chemotherapy recently was compared in the randomized phase 2 RTOG trial 0113. In this trial, a regimen of induction paclitaxel/5-FU/cisplatin followed by weekly paclitaxel/5-FU and radiation was compared with induction paclitaxel/cisplatin and weekly paclitaxel/cisplatin with radiation as definitive therapy in locally advanced disease.[66] Neither arm achieved the prespecified 1-year survival rate, although there appeared to be a nonsignificant trend toward improved survival in the 5-FU-containing arm (median OS 29 versus 15 months). Both arms also were associated with a grade 3/4 toxicity rate of greater than 80%. The authors concluded that neither arm was sufficiently superior to historical cisplatin/5-FU and radiation to warrant further investigation.

Docetaxel also has undergone more preliminary evaluation, as reported in phase 1/2 studies that have combined it with radiation and with cisplatin,[67] with 5-FU,[68] or with cisplatin/5-FU.[69] These studies have revealed an acceptable toxicity profile, consisting primarily of hematologic toxicities and mucositis. Although the other studies have not mandated surgery, the phase 2 evaluation of induction docetaxel/cisplatin followed by weekly docetaxel/cisplatin and radiation reported a near-complete and complete pathologic response in 48% of patients, with survival data comparable to other phase 2 evaluations.

In addition, oxaliplatin, a newer platinum analog, recently was evaluated in phase 1/2 studies that combined radiation with biweekly infusions of oxaliplatin and continuous infusion 5-FU.[70,71] The pCR rate was 25% to 38%. Toxicities were very manageable, with only 21% of patients in the preoperative group of the phase 2 study reporting grade 3 toxicities. The Southwest Oncology Group (SWOG) 0356 study is evaluating this regimen in a multicenter setting.

Finally, irinotecan-based regimens also have been investigated. A regimen of weekly irinotecan/cisplatin and radiation has been evaluated in phase 1 and 2 studies.[72–74] The regimen was found to be tolerable and is associated with pCR rates of 19% to 35%. Based on these positive results, the CALGB 80,302 trial is evaluating weekly irinotecan/cisplatin with concurrent radiation for locally advanced esophageal cancer.

The ECOG 1201 trial recently compared weekly irinotecan/cisplatin versus weekly paclitaxel/cisplatin, with concurrent radiation, followed by surgery and adjuvant therapy with the respective preoperative regimens in patients who had esophageal adenocarcinoma.[75] The results, presented in abstract form, revealed a disappointingly low pCR rate of 15% and 16% respectively, with a toxicity profile comparable to that historically noted with standard cisplatin/5-FU and radiation. These pCR rates, however, are within the range of 9% to 25% reported as the pCR rates for adenocarcinoma histology in the phase 3 trials of chemoradiotherapy described earlier. Median OS in the irinotecan/cisplatin arm is 34.9 months, while median OS in the paclitaxel/cisplatin arm is 21 months (with overlapping confidence intervals for both arms).[76] Based on these data, the authors conclude that neither regimen is clearly superior to conventional cisplatin/5-FU and radiation.

TARGETED THERAPIES

As with many other solid tumor malignancies, targeted therapies also have been the subject of intense interest. Although numerous such therapies have been investigated in phase 1/2 studies in both the locally advanced and metastatic setting, two large phase 3 trials for localized disease are underway. In the United Kingdom, the MAGIC-B trial is randomizing patients who have locally advanced gastric and GE junction cancer to peri-operative ECX chemotherapy (epirubicin/cisplatin/capecitabine) with or without bevacizumab, a monoclonal antibody against vascular endothelial growth factor. The RTOG 0436 trial is evaluating cisplatin/paclitaxel and radiation with or without cetuximab, a monoclonal antibody against epidermal growth factor receptor, in the nonoperative management of esophageal cancer.

POSITRON EMISSION TOMOGRAPHY-DIRECTED THERAPY

[18F]2-fluoro-deoxy-D-glucose positron emission tomography (FDG-PET) scanning is emerging as an important tool to investigate response to therapy. Several studies have demonstrated that the degree of response detected by PET following preoperative chemoradiotherapy[77,78] or chemotherapy[79,80] is correlated highly with pathologic response at surgery and with patient survival.

The German MUNICON trial evaluated the strategy of taking patients who had locally advanced GE junction tumors with a suboptimal response to 2 weeks of induction chemotherapy with cisplatin/5-FU—as determined by serial PET scans—directly to immediate surgery, instead of continuing with presumably ineffective chemotherapy. Patients who had a metabolic response by PET (defined as at least 35% reduction in standard uptake value between baseline and repeat PET scan) continued with an additional 12 weeks of chemotherapy before surgery.[81] This trial revealed a significantly improved R0 resection rate (96% versus 74%), major pathologic response rate (58% versus 0%), median event-free survival (29.7 versus 14.1 months), and median OS (median not reached versus 25.8 months) for PET responders versus PET nonresponders. The outcome for PET nonresponders referred for immediate surgery was similar to the outcome of such patients in an earlier trial who completed 3 months of preoperative chemotherapy,[79] indicating that nonresponding patients were not compromised by referral to immediate surgery.

Building on the results of the MUNICON trial, the same investigators recently reported the results of the MUNICON-2 trial in abstract form.[82] In this variant trial design, PET nonresponders to the same regimen of preoperative 5-FU/cisplatin were treated with salvage chemoradiotherapy with cisplatin before surgery. When compared with the PET responders who completed 3 months of 5-FU/cisplatin before surgery, the PET nonresponders had an inferior pCR rate (0% versus 16%), a higher R1/R2 resection rate (31% versus 16%), and an inferior 1-year PFS (46% versus 63%). These results are not entirely surprising, given the use of chemotherapy during concurrent radiation that was assessed to be suboptimal by PET when administered as induction therapy.

Based on the poor outcome of PET nonresponders in the previously mentioned study who proceeded directly to surgery, another possible strategy would be to use PET assessment after induction chemotherapy to dictate subsequent chemotherapy during concurrent radiation. Responding patients can continue with the same chemotherapy regimen during concurrent radiation, while nonresponding patients can be switched to alternative, noncross-resistant chemotherapy during radiation. Long-term disease-free survival has been reported in patients who progressed on induction chemotherapy but were changed to alternative chemotherapy during subsequent combined chemoradiotherapy.[74]

SUMMARY

The treatment of esophageal cancer remains a great challenge to medical, surgical, and radiation oncologists.

Nevertheless, recent trials indicate that more than surgery alone should be offered to patients. Primary chemoradiotherapy is now the standard of care in the treatment of inoperable, localized disease. The use of preoperative chemoradiotherapy continues to be investigated but appears to lead to an improvement in resectability and improved OS in patients who have had a pCR. Several recent trials have suggested that pre- or peri-operative chemotherapy is also a valid strategy in adenocarcinoma. The use of preoperative chemotherapy over chemoradiotherapy in SCC is supported less by the literature, given the equivocal phase 3 data and limited survival benefit seen in meta-analyses. For patients undergoing primary resection of lower esophageal and GE junction adenocarcinoma, postoperative chemoradiotherapy may improve survival compared with surgery alone.

Although surgery remains the standard curative treatment for early stage disease, there are data that definitive chemoradiotherapy results in similar survival rates as surgery alone. Similarly, definitive chemoradiotherapy is an accepted approach for patients who have SCC. Surgery for SCC patients who respond to initial chemoradiotherapy improves local control but does not impact clearly on survival. For patients who have locally persistent disease after chemoradiotherapy, surgery may remain a salvage option.

In contrast, the value of surgery for patients with adenocarcinoma who undergo initial chemoradiotherapy remains unanswered. Such patients, however, may experience benefit from surgery, based at least in part on the lower pCR rate observed after preoperative chemoradiotherapy for adenocarcinoma compared with SCC histology.

REFERENCES

1. Jemal A, Siegel R, Ward E, et al. Cancer statistics, 2008. CA Cancer J Clin 2008; 58:71–96.
2. Parkin DM, Bray F, Ferlay J, et al. Global cancer statistics, 2002. CA Cancer J Clin 2005;55:74–108.
3. Crew KD, Neugut AI. Epidemiology of upper gastrointestinal malignancies. Semin Oncol 2004;31:450–64.
4. Devesa SS, Fraumeni JF Jr. The rising incidence of gastric cardia cancer. J Natl Cancer Inst 1999;91:747–9.
5. Hulscher JB, van Sandick JW, de Boer AG, et al. Extended transthoracic resection compared with limited transhiatal resection for adenocarcinoma of the esophagus. N Engl J Med 2002;347:1662–9.
6. Muller JM, Erasmi H, Stelzner M, et al. Surgical therapy of oesophageal carcinoma. Br J Surg 1990;77:845–57.
7. Earlam R, Cunha-Melo JR. Oesophageal squamous cell carcinoma: I. A critical review of surgery. Br J Surg 1980;67:381–90.
8. Enzinger PC, Mayer RJ. Esophageal cancer. N Engl J Med 2003;349:2241–52.
9. Harris DT, Mastrangelo MJ. Theory and application of early systemic therapy. Semin Oncol 1991;18:493–503.
10. Kok T, Lanschot J, Siersema P, et al. Neoadjuvant chemotherapy in operable esophageal squamous cell cancer: final report of a phase III multicenter randomized controlled trial [abstract 984]. In: Proceedings of American Society of Clinical Oncology Annual Meeting. 1997.
11. Kelsen DP, Ginsberg R, Pajak TF, et al. Chemotherapy followed by surgery compared with surgery alone for localized esophageal cancer. N Engl J Med 1998;339:1979–84.
12. Medical Research Council Oesophageal Cancer Working Group. Surgical resection with or without preoperative chemotherapy in oesophageal cancer: a randomised controlled trial. Lancet 2002;359:1727–33.
13. Allum W, Fogarty P, Stenning S, et al. Long-term results of the MRC OEO2 randomized trial of surgery with or without preoperative chemotherapy in

resectable esophageal cancer. [abstract 9]. In: Proceedings of the Gastrointestinal Cancers Symposium. Orlando (FL). 2008.

14. Gebski V, Burmeister B, Smithers BM, et al. Survival benefits from neoadjuvant chemoradiotherapy or chemotherapy in oesophageal carcinoma: a meta-analysis. Lancet Oncol 2007;8:226–34.

15. Thirion P, Michiels S, Le Maître A, et al. Individual patient data-based meta-analysis assessing preoperative chemotherapy in resectable oesophageal carcinoma [abstract 4512]. In: Proceedings of American Society of Clinical Oncology Annual Meeting. Chicago. 2007.

16. Cunningham D, Allum WH, Stenning SP, et al. Perioperative chemotherapy versus surgery alone for resectable gastroesophageal cancer. N Engl J Med 2006;355: 11–20.

17. Boige V, Pignon J, Saint-Aubert B, et al. Final results of a randomized trial comparing preoperative 5-fluorouracil (F)/cisplatin (P) to surgery alone in adenocarcinoma of stomach and lower esophagus (ASLE): FNLCC ACCORD07-FFCD 9703 trial [abstract 4510]. In: Proceedings of American Society of Clinical Oncology Annual Meeting. Chicago. 2007.

18. Kelsen DP, Minsky B, Smith M, et al. Preoperative therapy for esophageal cancer: a randomized comparison of chemotherapy versus radiation therapy. J Clin Oncol 1990;8:1352–61.

19. Arnott SJ, Duncan W, Kerr GR, et al. Low-dose preoperative radiotherapy for carcinoma of the oesophagus: results of a randomized clinical trial. Radiother Oncol 1992;24:108–13.

20. Nygaard K, Hagen S, Hansen HS, et al. Preoperative radiotherapy prolongs survival in operable esophageal carcinoma: a randomized, multicenter study of pre-operative radiotherapy and chemotherapy. The second Scandinavian trial in esophageal cancer. World J Surg 1992;16:1104–9.

21. Arnott SJ, Duncan W, Gignoux M, et al. Preoperative radiotherapy for esophageal carcinoma. Cochrane Database Syst Rev 2005;CD001799.

22. Ando N, Iizuka T, Kakegawa T, et al. A randomized trial of surgery with and without chemotherapy for localized squamous carcinoma of the thoracic esophagus: the Japan Clinical Oncology Group Study. J Thorac Cardiovasc Surg 1997; 114:205–9.

23. Ando N, Iizuka T, Ide H, et al. Surgery plus chemotherapy compared with surgery alone for localized squamous cell carcinoma of the thoracic esophagus: a Japan Clinical Oncology Group Study–JCOG9204. J Clin Oncol 2003;21:4592–6.

24. Igaki H, Kato H, Ando N, et al. A randomized trial of postoperative adjuvant chemotherapy with cisplatin and 5-fluorouracil versus neoadjuvant chemotherapy for clinical stage II/III squamous cell carcinoma of the thoracic esophagus (JCOG 9907) [abstract 4510]. In: Proceedings of American Society of Clinical Oncology Annual Meeting. Chicago. 2008.

25. Pouliquen X, Levard H, Hay JM, et al. 5-Fluorouracil and cisplatin therapy after palliative surgical resection of squamous cell carcinoma of the esophagus. A multicenter randomized trial. French Associations for Surgical Research. Ann Surg 1996;223:127–33.

26. Armanios M, Xu R, Forastiere AA, et al. Adjuvant chemotherapy for resected adenocarcinoma of the esophagus, gastro–esophageal junction, and cardia: phase II trial (E8296) of the Eastern Cooperative Oncology Group. J Clin Oncol 2004;22:4495–9.

27. Teniere P, Hay JM, Fingerhut A, et al. Postoperative radiation therapy does not increase survival after curative resection for squamous cell carcinoma of the middle

and lower esophagus as shown by a multicenter controlled trial. French University Association for Surgical Research. Surg Gynecol Obstet 1991;173:123–30.

28. Fok M, Sham JS, Choy D, et al. Postoperative radiotherapy for carcinoma of the esophagus: a prospective, randomized controlled study. Surgery 1993;113:138–47.

29. Xiao ZF, Yang ZY, Liang J, et al. Value of radiotherapy after radical surgery for esophageal carcinoma: a report of 495 patients. Ann Thorac Surg 2003;75:331–6.

30. Macdonald JS, Smalley SR, Benedetti J, et al. Chemoradiotherapy after surgery compared with surgery alone for adenocarcinoma of the stomach or gastro-esophageal junction. N Engl J Med 2001;345:725–30.

31. Coia LR, Engstrom PF, Paul AR, et al. Long-term results of infusional 5-FU, mitomycin-C and radiation as primary management of esophageal carcinoma. Int J Radiat Oncol Biol Phys 1991;20:29–36.

32. Valerdi JJ, Tejedor M, Illarramendi JJ, et al. Neoadjuvant chemotherapy and radiotherapy in locally advanced esophagus carcinoma: long-term results. Int J Radiat Oncol Biol Phys 1993;27:843–7.

33. Berger AC, Farma J, Scott WJ, et al. Complete response to neoadjuvant chemo-radiotherapy in esophageal carcinoma is associated with significantly improved survival. J Clin Oncol 2005;23:4330–7.

34. Forastiere AA, Orringer MB, Perez-Tamayo C, et al. Preoperative chemoradiation followed by transhiatal esophagectomy for carcinoma of the esophagus: final report. J Clin Oncol 1993;11:1118–23.

35. Heath EI, Burtness BA, Heitmiller RF, et al. Phase II evaluation of preoperative chemoradiation and postoperative adjuvant chemotherapy for squamous cell and adenocarcinoma of the esophagus. J Clin Oncol 2000;18:868–76.

36. Makary MA, Kiernan PD, Sheridan MJ, et al. Multimodality treatment for esophageal cancer: the role of surgery and neoadjuvant therapy. Am Surg 2003;69:693–700.

37. Stahl M, Stuschke M, Lehmann N, et al. Chemoradiation with and without surgery in patients with locally advanced squamous cell carcinoma of the esophagus. J Clin Oncol 2005;23:2310–7.

38. Geh JI. The use of chemoradiotherapy in oesophageal cancer. Eur J Cancer 2002;38:300–13.

39. Herskovic A, Martz K, al-Sarraf M, et al. Combined chemotherapy and radio-therapy compared with radiotherapy alone in patients with cancer of the esophagus. N Engl J Med 1992;326:1593–8.

40. Cooper JS, Guo MD, Herskovic A, et al. Chemoradiotherapy of locally advanced esophageal cancer: long-term follow-up of a prospective randomized trial (RTOG 85-01). Radiation Therapy Oncology Group. JAMA 1999;281:1623–7.

41. Minsky BD, Neuberg D, Kelsen DP, et al. Final report of Intergroup Trial 0122 (ECOG PE-289, RTOG 90-12): phase II trial of neoadjuvant chemotherapy plus concurrent chemotherapy and high-dose radiation for squamous cell carcinoma of the esophagus. Int J Radiat Oncol Biol Phys 1999;43:517–23.

42. Minsky BD, Pajak TF, Ginsberg RJ, et al. INT 0123 (Radiation Therapy Oncology Group 94-05) phase III trial of combined-modality therapy for esophageal cancer: high-dose versus standard-dose radiation therapy. J Clin Oncol 2002;20:1167–74.

43. Gaspar LE, Winter K, Kocha WI, et al. A phase I/II study of external beam radia-tion, brachytherapy, and concurrent chemotherapy for patients with localized carcinoma of the esophagus (Radiation Therapy Oncology Group Study 9207): final report. Cancer 2000;88:988–95.

44. Urba SG, Orringer MB, Turrisi A, et al. Randomized trial of preoperative chemo-radiation versus surgery alone in patients with locoregional esophageal carci-noma. J Clin Oncol 2001;19:305–13.

45. Walsh TN, Noonan N, Hollywood D, et al. A comparison of multimodal therapy and surgery for esophageal adenocarcinoma. N Engl J Med 1996;335:462.

46. Orringer MB, Marshall B, Iannettoni MD. Transhiatal esophagectomy: clinical experience and refinements. Ann Surg 1999;230:392–400.

47. Bosset JF, Gignoux M, Triboulet JP, et al. Chemoradiotherapy followed by surgery compared with surgery alone in squamous-cell cancer of the esophagus. N Engl J Med 1997;337:161–7.

48. Burmeister BH, Smithers BM, Gebski V, et al. Surgery alone versus chemoradiotherapy followed by surgery for resectable cancer of the oesophagus: a randomised controlled phase III trial. Lancet Oncol 2005;6:659–68.

49. Tepper J, Krasna MJ, Niedzwiecki D, et al. Phase III trial of trimodality therapy with cisplatin, fluorouracil, radiotherapy, and surgery compared with surgery alone for esophageal cancer: CALGB 9781. J Clin Oncol 2008;26:1086–92.

50. Stahl M, Walz M, Stuschke M, et al. Preoperative chemotherapy (CTX) versus preoperative chemoradiotherapy (CRTX) in locally advanced esophagogastric adenocarcinomas: first results of a randomized phase III trial [abstract 4511]. In: Proceedings of American Society of Clinical Oncology Annual Meeting. Chicago. 2007.

51. Stahl M, Wilke H, Lehmann N, et al. Long-term results of a phase III study investigating chemoradiation with and without surgery in locally advanced squamous cell carcinoma (LA-SCC) of the esophagus [abstract 4530]. In: Proceedings of American Society of Clinical Oncology Annual Meeting. Chicago. 2008.

52. Bedenne L, Michel P, Bouche O, et al. Chemoradiation followed by surgery compared with chemoradiation alone in squamous cancer of the esophagus: FFCD 9102. J Clin Oncol 2007;25:1160–8.

53. Jouve J, Michel P, Mariette C, et al. Outcome of the nonrandomized patients in the FFCD 9102 trial: chemoradiation followed by surgery compared with chemoradiation alone in squamous cancer of the esophagus [abstract 4555]. In: Proceedings of American Society of Clinical Oncology Annual Meeting. Chicago. 2007.

54. Carstens H, Albertsson M, Friesland S, et al. A randomized trial of chemoradiotherapy versus surgery alone in patients with resectable esophageal cancer [abstract 4530]. In: Proceedings of American Society of Clinical Oncology Annual Meeting. Chicago. 2007.

55. Adelstein DJ, Rice TW, Rybicki LA, et al. Does paclitaxel improve the chemoradiotherapy of locoregionally advanced esophageal cancer? A nonrandomized comparison with fluorouracil-based therapy. J Clin Oncol 2000;18:2032–9.

56. Blanke CD, Choy H, Teng M, et al. Concurrent paclitaxel and thoracic irradiation for locally advanced esophageal cancer. Semin Radiat Oncol 1999;9:43–52.

57. Urba SG, Orringer MB, Ianettonni M, et al. Concurrent cisplatin, paclitaxel, and radiotherapy as preoperative treatment for patients with locoregional esophageal carcinoma. Cancer 2003;98:2177–83.

58. Brenner B, Ilson DH, Minsky BD, et al. Phase I trial of combined-modality therapy for localized esophageal cancer: escalating doses of continuous-infusion paclitaxel with cisplatin and concurrent radiation therapy. J Clin Oncol 2004;22:45–52.

59. Safran H, Gaissert H, Akerman P, et al. Paclitaxel, cisplatin, and concurrent radiation for esophageal cancer. Cancer Invest 2001;19:1–7.

60. van Meerten E, Muller K, Tilanus HW, et al. Neoadjuvant concurrent chemoradiation with weekly paclitaxel and carboplatin for patients with oesophageal cancer: a phase II study. Br J Cancer 2006;94:1389–94.

61. Henry LR, Goldberg M, Scott W, et al. Induction cisplatin and paclitaxel followed by combination chemoradiotherapy with 5-fluorouracil, cisplatin, and paclitaxel

before resection in localized esophageal cancer: a phase II report. Ann Surg Oncol 2006;13:214–20.

62. Meluch AA, Greco FA, Gray JR, et al. Preoperative therapy with concurrent paclitaxel/carboplatin/infusional 5-FU and radiation therapy in locoregional esophageal cancer: final results of a Minnie Pearl Cancer Research Network phase II trial. Cancer J 2003;9:251–60.

63. Weiner LM, Colarusso P, Goldberg M, et al. Combined-modality therapy for esophageal cancer: phase I trial of escalating doses of paclitaxel in combination with cisplatin, 5-fluorouracil, and high-dose radiation before esophagectomy. Semin Oncol 1997;24:S19–93.

64. Wright CD, Wain JC, Lynch TJ, et al. Induction therapy for esophageal cancer with paclitaxel and hyperfractionated radiotherapy: a phase I and II study. J Thorac Cardiovasc Surg 1997;114:811–5.

65. Roof KS, Coen J, Lynch TJ, et al. Concurrent cisplatin, 5-FU, paclitaxel, and radiation therapy in patients with locally advanced esophageal cancer. Int J Radiat Oncol Biol Phys 2006;65:1120–8.

66. Ajani JA, Winter K, Komaki R, et al. Phase II randomized trial of two nonoperative regimens of induction chemotherapy followed by chemoradiation in patients with localized carcinoma of the esophagus: RTOG 0113. J Clin Oncol 2008;26:4551–6.

67. Schuller J, Balmer-Majno S, Mingrone W, et al. Preoperative induction chemotherapy with docetaxel-cisplatin followed by concurrent docetaxel-cisplatin and radiation therapy (RT) in patients with locally advanced esophageal cancer: final results of the multicenter phase II trial SAKK 75/02 [abstract 4550]. In: Proceedings of American Society of Clinical Oncology Annual Meeting. Chicago. 2008.

68. Hihara J, Yoshida K, Hamai Y, et al. Phase I study of docetaxel (TXT) and 5-fluorouracil (5-FU) with concurrent radiotherapy in patients with advanced esophageal cancer. Anticancer Res 2007;27:2597–603.

69. Higuchi K, Koizumi W, Tanabe S, et al. A phase I trial of definitive chemoradiotherapy with docetaxel, cisplatin, and 5-fluorouracil (DCF-R) for advanced esophageal carcinoma: Kitasato digestive disease & oncology group trial (KDOG 0501). Radiother Oncol 2008;87:398–404.

70. Khushalani NI, Leichman CG, Proulx G, et al. Oxaliplatin in combination with protracted-infusion fluorouracil and radiation: report of a clinical trial for patients with esophageal cancer. J Clin Oncol 2002;20:2844–50.

71. O'Connor BM, Chadha MK, Pande A, et al. Concurrent oxaliplatin, 5-fluorouracil, and radiotherapy in the treatment of locally advanced esophageal carcinoma. Cancer J 2007;13:119–24.

72. Enzinger P, Mamon H, Choi N, et al. Phase II cisplatin, irinotecan, celecoxib, and concurrent radiation therapy followed by surgery for locally advanced esophageal cancer [abstract 35]. In: Proceedings of Gastrointestinal Cancers Symposium. San Francisco (CA). 2004.

73. Ilson DH, Bains M, Kelsen DP, et al. Phase I trial of escalating-dose irinotecan given weekly with cisplatin and concurrent radiotherapy in locally advanced esophageal cancer. J Clin Oncol 2003;21:2926–32.

74. Ku G, Bains M, Rizk N, et al. Phase II trial of preoperative cisplatin/irinotecan and radiotherapy for locally advanced esophageal cancer: PET scan after induction therapy may identify early treatment failure [abstract 9]. In: Proceedings of Gastrointestinal Cancers Symposium. Orlando (FL). 2007.

75. Kleinberg L, Powell M, Forastiere A, et al. E1201: an Eastern Cooperative Oncology Group (ECOG) randomized phase II trial of neoadjuvant preoperative paclitaxel/cisplatin/RT or irinotecan/cisplatin/RT in endoscopy with ultrasound

(EUS) staged adenocarcinoma of the esophagus [abstract 4533]. In: Proceedings of American Society of Clinical Oncology Annual Meeting. Chicago. 2007.

76. Kleinberg L, Powell M, Forastiere A, et al. Survival outcome of E1201: an Eastern Cooperative Oncology Group (ECOG) randomized phase II trial of neoadjuvant preoperative paclitaxel/cisplatin/radiotherapy (RT) or irinotecan/cisplatin/RT in endoscopy with ultrasound (EUS) staged esophageal adenocarcinoma [abstract 4532]. In: Proceedings of American Society of Clinical Oncology Annual Meeting. Chicago. 2008.

77. Downey RJ, Akhurst T, Ilson D, et al. Whole body 18FDG-PET and the response of esophageal cancer to induction therapy: results of a prospective trial. J Clin Oncol 2003;21:428–32.

78. Flamen P, Van Cutsem E, Lerut A, et al. Positron emission tomography for assessment of the response to induction radiochemotherapy in locally advanced oesophageal cancer. Ann Oncol 2002;13:361–8.

79. Ott K, Weber WA, Lordick F, et al. Metabolic imaging predicts response, survival, and recurrence in adenocarcinomas of the esophagogastric junction. J Clin Oncol 2006;24:4692–8.

80. Weber WA, Ott K, Becker K, et al. Prediction of response to preoperative chemotherapy in adenocarcinomas of the esophagogastric junction by metabolic imaging. J Clin Oncol 2001;19:3058–65.

81. Lordick F, Ott K, Krause BJ, et al. PET to assess early metabolic response and to guide treatment of adenocarcinoma of the oesophagogastric junction: the MUNICON phase II trial. Lancet Oncol 2007;8:797–805.

82. Lordick F, Ott K, Krause B, et al. Salvage radiochemotherapy in locally advanced gastroesophageal junction tumors that are metabolically resistant to induction chemotherapy: the MUNICON-2 trial [abstract 104]. In: Proceedings of Gastrointestinal Cancers Symposium. Orlando (FL). 2008.

Traditional Chinese Medicinal Herbs in the Treatment of Patients with Esophageal Cancer: A Systematic Review

Taixiang Wu, MD[a],*, Xunzhe Yang, MSc[a], Xiaoxi Zeng, MSc[a],
Guy D. Eslick, PhD, MMedSc (Clin Epi), MMedStat[b]

KEYWORDS

- Esophageal cancer • Traditional Chinese medicine
- Treatment • Effect • Systematic review

Esophageal cancer is the seventh leading cause of cancer death worldwide. It has two subtypes—squamous carcinoma and adenocarcinoma. The occurrence of esophageal cancer varies by geographic area, ethnic group, and gender. The incidence of esophageal cancer in particular areas of northern Iran is as high as 30 to 800 cases per 100,000 persons and in some areas of southern Russia, northern China, and the United States approximately three to six cases per 100,000 persons.[1,2] It is generally more common in men than in women; the incidence in males is seven times higher than in females.[3,4]

Esophageal cancer is highly treatable by surgery in its earliest stages but is usually fatal in the advanced stages.[5,6] The application of treatment is dependent on the stage of the disease at diagnosis. Esophageal resection (esophagectomy) is used in patients who are suitable for surgery. Nonoperative therapy is usually reserved for patients who are not candidates for surgery. The goal of therapy for these patients is palliation of dysphagia. Chemotherapy, radiotherapy, or both are used to relieve dysphagia for these patients, to kill possible residual cancer cells in postoperative cases, and to limit the cancer in patients with advanced esophageal cancer as preoperative treatment.[7,8]

Chinese medicinal herbs have commonly been used as an adjunct treatment for alleviating the side effects of chemotherapy or radiotherapy and for improving the

[a] Chinese Cochrane Centre, Chinese EBM Centre, West China Hospital, Sichuan University, Chengdu, China
[b] School of Public Health, The University of Sydney, Sydney, Australia
* Corresponding author.
E-mail address: txwutx@hotmail.com (T. Wu).

Gastroenterol Clin N Am 38 (2009) 153–167
doi:10.1016/j.gtc.2009.01.006
0889-8553/09/$ – see front matter © 2009 Elsevier Inc. All rights reserved.

quality of life of esophageal cancer patients. Possible benefits of herbal medicines include increasing appetite, boosting the immune system,[9] facilitating the recovery of the body, and preventing tumor regeneration or the development of metastases.[10] A Cochrane systematic review including two trials suggested that Zhenxiang capsules or Huachansu injection may not improve the effects of short-term therapy or the 1-year survival rate when used as an adjunct to chemo- or radiotherapy in the treatment of esophageal cancer. The quality of life may be improved by Huachansu injection; however, the evidence was weak due to the poor quality of these two studies.[11] The purpose of this article was to review publications to assess the efficacy and possible adverse effects of Chinese medicinal herbs integrated with chemo- or radiotherapy for the treatment of esophageal cancer.

METHODS
Criteria for Considering Studies for this Review

Randomized controlled trials referring to the clinical utility and safety of the administration of traditional Chinese medicines (TCM) in any form, for example, oral decoction, intravenous, or gastrogavage, for the treatment of esophageal cancer as an adjunct to active cancer therapy such as radiotherapy or chemotherapy were considered as eligible for inclusion. The comparator could be active therapy without TCM or placebo. Patients with different subtypes at any stage of esophageal cancer were eligible for inclusion.

Outcomes

Outcomes reviewed included the following:
  Mortality or median survival times
  Time to progression
  Quality of life, include reducing gastrointestinal tract symptoms and other adverse
    reactions caused by radiochemotherapy
  Improvement of disease, defined as a complete response and partial response as
    clarified by Miller,[12] or short-term therapeutic effects
  Immune function as defined by T-lymph cell subsets
  Adverse events, defined as any adverse event resulting from TCM that caused
    death,[1] life-threatening illness,[2] or significant toxicity[3]

Search Methods for Identification of Studies

We searched electronic databases using the terms *esophageal cancer* and *Chinese herbs* or *traditional Chinese medicine* or *Chinese medicinal herbs*. Trials were identified by searching the following electronic databases up to September of 2008: the CENTRAL database of the Cochrane Library (issue 2, 2008), MEDLINE, the Chinese Biomedical Database, the China National Knowledge Infrastructure, the VIP database, and the WANFANG database.

Data Collection and Analysis

The study selection was undertaken by two reviewers (YXZ and WTX).

Selection of Studies

Full articles of studies that mentioned "randomly allocated patients" were retrieved for further assessment. At first, the authors of potential included studies were telephoned to determine whether they were randomized controlled trials. There were no recorded disagreements between reviewers.

Data Extraction

Data extracted from each of the included studies concerned the details of the study population, the type and stage of esophageal cancer, the duration and dosing schedule of interventions, outcomes, and any treatment-related adverse events observed. Methods and quality issues were also extracted (eg, the design, duration of follow-up, method of randomization, allocation concealment, and blinding).

Assessment of Potential Risk of Bias of Included Studies

Several characteristics were assessed according to the quality standard previously described by Wu and Liu.[13]

Randomization process

A. A random number table or computer software used to generate random numbers was judged as an adequate procedure of randomization. Coin tossing or shuffling used for generating the random allocation sequence before the trial launching was considered eligible and associated with a low risk of selection bias.

B. A study that did not specify one of the adequate methods outlined previously but only mentioned "random" was considered to have a moderate risk of selection bias.

C. Other methods of allocation (eg, quasi-randomization) or that optionally allocated the patients that appeared to have a high risk of bias were excluded.

Allocation concealment process

A. Measures to conceal allocation were defined as adequate when the person who generated an allocation sequence did not intend to recruit the participants (eg, central randomization) and when the allocation sequences were conserved safely by special persons (eg, sealed in opaque envelopes or kept in a secured computer) or another description was used that contained convincing elements of concealment. These measures were considered to have a low risk of selection bias.

B. Concealed trials in which the author did not report an approach of allocation concealment at all were considered as having a moderate risk of selection bias.

C. Inadequate allocation concealment was defined as an approach that did not fall into one of the categories in A.

D. The study did not conceal allocation.

Methods C and D were considered as having a high risk of selection bias.

Level of blinding

A. In double or triple blinding, the health care provider, participants, and results assessor were masked. These studies were considered as having a low risk of performance and detection bias.

B. Single blinding of the results assessor was considered to have a moderate risk of performance and detection bias. If single blinding of the patients but not of the results assessor was performed, the study was considered to have a high risk of detection bias.

C. Nonblinding was considered to have a high risk of performance and detection bias.

There was no bias for assessment of mortality whether blinded or not.

Incomplete outcome data
A. There was a low risk of bias in trials in which few drop-out/losses to follow-up were noted and an intention-to-treat analysis was possible.
B. There was a moderate risk of bias in trials reporting that the rate of exclusion was about 10%, regardless of whether intention-to-treat analysis was used.
C. There was a high risk of bias when the rate of exclusion was at least 15%, or when wide differences in exclusions between groups occurred, regardless of whether intention-to-treat analysis was used.

Selective report
No. There was a low risk of reporting bias. All of the outcomes were reported in detail.

Probably yes. There was a moderate risk of reporting bias. At least one of outcomes was mentioned but not in detail.

Yes. There was a high risk of reporting bias. At least one of the outcomes was not reported.

Measures of Treatment Effects

Due to the differences in the formulas used in the included studies, we did not perform combined analysis. The effects of dichotomous data were measured as relative risk (RR) with a 95% confidence interval (CI). Continuous data as were presented as a mean difference (MD) with a 95% CI.

RESULTS
Description of Studies

Results of the search
The initial search of the electronic databases yielded 8 studies in CENTRAL, 112 in PubMed, 2755 in the Chinese National Knowledge Infrastructure, 1271 in VIP, and 53 in WANFANG. After scrutinizing these studies, 127 studies mentioning "randomly allocated patients" were identified. All of these studies were conducted in China. A total of 119 authors of these studies were contacted by telephone, and the studies were identified as nonrandomized controlled trials and therefore excluded. One study obtained outcomes that did not match our inclusion criteria and was also excluded.[14]

The author of a published study that included 40 patients[15] was communicated with by telephone. The author stated that the study currently included 100 patients and that the data were being analyzed. We considered this to be an incomplete study and decided to classify it as an ongoing study.

One study was duplicated three times.[16-18] We decided to abstract data from the first version.[16] The authors of these three reports and other authors of four studies[19-22] could not be contacted by telephone to confirm the randomization method used and other quality issues. Nevertheless, we included these studies in the review because they were performed in high-level hospitals and could be representative of TCM used in the treatment of esophageal cancer. The flowchart of included studies is shown in **Fig. 1.**

Characteristics of included studies
Design Four studies[19-22] had two parallel arms and one had three.[16] "Randomly allocated patients" were mentioned.

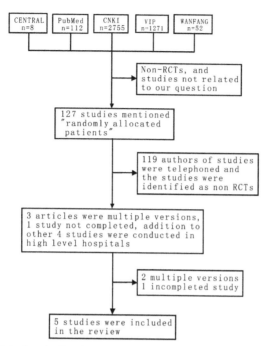

Fig. 1. Flowchart of study selection.

Studied populations A total of 406 esophageal cancer patients were included from five studies. Two studies[16,19] included postoperative patients; the others included advanced esophageal cancer patients.

Interventions

In three studies,[19,20,22] chemo- or radiotherapy or both were given to both groups. In addition to chemo- or radiotherapy, TCM decoction was given to TCM group patients orally. The contents of TCM decoctions were modified according to different TCM signs. The modified traditional TCM formula Sijunzi Tang decoction,[19] Liuwei Dihuan Wan decoction,[20] and self-prepared formula[22] were adjunctively used during the radio- or chemotherapy, respectively.

In one study, one group received standard chemotherapy, one group received a TCM decoction prepared by authors themselves according to the signs of patients for 12 months, and one group received both chemotherapy and an oral TCM decoction for 12 months.[16] The contents of TCM preparations are listed in **Table 1**.

OUTCOMES

One study[19] reported rates of mortality and survival; one study[20] assessed the T-lymph cell subsets count, tumor necrosis factor alpha (TNF-alpha), radiation esophagitis, and change of Karnofsky scores; one study[21] assessed the T-lymph cell subsets count; one study[16] reported the recurrence of tumor or metastasis, survival rate, immune function including cellular and humoral immunity, and quality of life; and one study[22] assessed the acute esophageal toxic reaction.

Table 1 Essential contents of TCM preparations			
Preparation	Pinyin Name	Latin Name	English Name
Liuwei Dihuang Wan			
	Shu Dihuang	*Radix rehmanniae*	Rehmannia root
	Shanzhuyu	*Fructus corni*	Common macrocarpium fruit
	Shanyao	*Rhizoma diosscoreae*	Common yam rhizome
	Mudanpi	*Cortex moutan*	Tree peony bark
	Fuling	*Poria*	Indian buead
	Zexie	*Rhizoma alismatis*	Oriental waterplantain rhizoma
Sijunzi Tang decoction			
	Renshen	*Radix ginseng*	Ginseng
	Fuling	*Poria*	Indian buead
	Baizhu	*Rhizoma atractylodis macrocephalae*	Largehead atractylodes rhizome
	Gancao	*Radix glycyrrhizae*	Liquoric root

Risk of Bias in Included Studies

All five studies did not describe the randomization methods used, although "randomly allocated patients" was mentioned. Moreover, no study mentioned allocation concealment; therefore, there was a high risk of selection bias in the included studies. Blinding was not used for results assessment in all included studies. Patients and trial staff had not been blinded because blinding the use of TCM decoction is very difficult. There was high risk of performance bias and detection bias in detecting subjective outcomes such as quality of life, Karnofsky scores, and so on.

Basically, each study reported the results in detail and completely, except the report of short-term effect in one study.[22] That study failed to define "short-term effect." We were unable to check whether all of the outcomes had been selectively reported or not. The characteristics of included studies are shown in **Table 2**.

Effects of Interventions

Mortality or survival times

One study[19] reported the mortality and survival rate of patients. In the first 2 years, 16 patients died in the TCM group and 24 died in the control group. There was no statistically significant difference between the two groups (RR = 0.46; 95% CI, 0.20–1.05). At the end of the fifth year after treatment, 36 patients in the TCM group versus 44 in the control group had died. There was a statistically significant difference (RR = 0.14; 95% CI, 0.03–0.65). The results show that giving a modified Sijunzi Tang decoction to postoperative esophageal cancer patients resulted in greater numbers of patients surviving until the fifth year after treatment.

One study[16] reported the number of survivors. There were 31 patients alive in the chemotherapy plus TCM group with a 72.1% survival rate after the first year of treatment compared with 20 (46.5%) in the chemotherapy group and 18 (42.9%) in the TCM group. There were statistically significant differences when comparing the chemotherapy plus TCM group versus the other two groups (RR = 1.55; 95% CI, 1.07–2.25 and RR = 1.68; 95% CI, 1.13–2.50, respectively). Similarly, the 2-year survival also showed a statistically significant difference. A total of 24 patients were alive in the chemotherapy plus TCM group compared with 12 survivors each in the other two groups (RR = 2.00; 95% CI, 1.15–3.46 and RR = 1.95; 95% CI, 1.13–3.38, respectively). These findings suggest that there are more postoperative esophageal cancer patients alive who take TCM decoction with chemotherapy than those treated by chemotherapy or TCM decoction alone. Although there was no statistically significant difference in survival at 3 years, there were more survivors in the chemotherapy plus TCM group when compared with the other two groups (16 versus 10 and 11, respectively) (RR = 1.60; 95% CI, 0.82–3.12 and RR = 1.42; 95% CI, 0.75–2.69, respectively). When compared with chemotherapy alone, TCM alone had no statistically significant difference in survival at 1 year (RR = 1.09; 95% CI, 0.68–1.74), 2 years (RR = 0.98; 95% CI, 0.50–1.92), or 3 years (RR = 0.89; 95% CI, 0.42–1.87).

Time to progression
None of studies reported the time to progression.

Quality of life
One study[16] reported the quality of life of esophageal cancer patients undergoing therapy. More patients in the chemotherapy plus TCM group had an improved quality of life when compared with those in the chemotherapy group; however, this difference was not statistically significant (25 versus 16) (RR = 1.56; 95% CI, 0.98–2.48), and a similar finding was found for the TCM group (25 versus 29) (RR = 0.84; 95% CI, 0.61–1.16). There was a statistically significant difference when comparing the TCM group with the chemotherapy group (RR = 0.54; 95% CI, 0.35–0.83), suggesting that the improvement of quality of life in the chemotherapy group was much less than in the TCM group. TCM decoction obviously improved the quality of life of postoperative esophageal cancer patients. Two studies[20,22] reported a reduction of adverse reactions of radiochemotherapy. Both suggested that the integrated use of TCM with radiochemotherapy reduced the number of and severity of adverse reactions, including digestive tract symptoms and improved physical power, but was not superior to the control in the prevalence of marrow inhibition.

Improvement of cancer, rate of relapse, or metastasis of cancer
One study[22] reported the "short-term efficacy" of treating cancer, but the data were unusable. Another study[16] reported that 30 of 42 patients in the TCM group, 33 of 43 in the chemotherapy group, and 23 of 43 in the chemotherapy plus TCM group appeared to relapse or develop cancer metastasis. The integrated use of TCM with chemotherapy showed a statistically lower incidence of relapse or metastasis of cancer than chemotherapy (RR = 0.35; 95% CI, 0.14–0.88), whereas TCM alone versus integrated TCM with chemotherapy and TCM alone versus chemotherapy did not show a statistically significant difference (RR = 0.46; 95% CI, 0.19–1.13 and RR = 0.76; 95% CI, 0.29–2.01, respectively).

Immune function
One study[20] detected the change of TNF-alpha levels. There was no significant difference between two groups (MD = 89.30; 95% CI, 6.39–204.99), suggesting that giving Liuwei Dihuang Tang decoction did not increase the TNF-alpha concentration. On the other hand, a comparison of the difference in CD4/CD8 before and after treatment appeared to show a statistically significant difference (MD = 0.34; 95% CI, 0.07–0.62), suggesting that the cellular immune function was increased after treatment with the Liuwei Dihuang Tang decoction. In addition, another study[21] reported that CD3 and CD4 concentrations increased (MD = 5.38; 95% CI, 1.00–9.76 and MD = 4.96; 95% CI, 1.41–8.51, respectively) and CD8 concentrations decreased (MD =

Table 2
Characteristics of included studies

Study	Method	Patients	Interventions	Outcomes
Cui 2006[19]	Parallel group "Envelope method of randomization" mentioned, but lack of detailed information of the randomization procedure	Postoperative participants (6 weeks after operation) identified as having phase II-III squamous epithelioma by histopathology with normal liver, renal function, and white cell count, without other severe disease Karnofsky scores >80, age <75 years included 48 in chemo- radiotherapy group, 46 in radio- and chemotherapy group	Both groups used same chemoradiotherapy courses: 5-FU, 750 mg/m^2 (day 1–5); DDP, 70 mg/m^2 (day 1): two courses (6-week interval between two courses) After two courses of chemotherapy, radiotherapy by 6 MV x-ray, 1 time daily, 2 Gy, 5 time/week, total 6 weeks Participants in TCM group given modified Sijunzi Tang decoction	Mortality, survival
Du 2006[20]	Parallel design Randomization mentioned as "lotting method" No blinding	A total of 30 patients in TCM group (20 male, 10 female); 30 in control group (22 male, 8 female) Age and disease condition similar	Radiotherapy same in both groups: 6 MV x-ray, 2 Gy/time, 5 times/week; DT 64–66 Gy for radical treatment, DT 50 Gy for palliative treatment Participants in TCM group given modified Liuwei Dihuang Wan decoction from day 3 before radiotherapy, one Ji daily, and administrated half dose in morning and evening, respectively, until completion of radiotherapy	T-lymph cell subsets count, including CD4, CD8, rate of CD4/CD8 TNF-alpha Radiation esophagitis Karnofsky scores

Gao 2006[21]	Parallel design "Randomly allocated patients" mentioned but lack of description about randomization process No blinding	A total of 54 participants diagnosed as having esophageal squamous epithelioma by histopathology 36 in TCM group (21 male, 15 female; average age, 54.8 years); 18 in control group (10 male, 8 female; average age, 57.5 years) All participants scheduled for a radical operation for esophageal cancer	Participants in TCM group given Huangqi Zengmian Shan 1 week before operation and not in the perioperative period; from day 8 after operation, given 4 weeks of TCM treatment Other therapy same as control group (not mentioned in detail)	T-lymph cell subsets: CD3, —D4, CD8, CD4/CD8
Li 2005[16]	Parallel design Random number table used to allocate participants Blinding performed	A total of 128 postoperative esophageal cancer patients: (1) 2–4 weeks after operation; (2) did not receive anti-tumor and immunologic treatment during the past month, Karnofsky scores >70; (3) without cancer metastasis 42 participants allocated to TCM group, 43 in TCM + chemotherapy group, and 43 in chemotherapy group	TCM group: herbal medicine only, basic formula modified according to the different Zheng of patients Chemotherapy group: 5-FU + cisplatin + calcium folinate + megestrol acetate tablets TCM + chemotherapy group: TCM same as TCM group, and chemotherapy same as chemotherapy group	Recurrence of tumor or metastasis Survival Immune function: T-lymph cell subsets, IgG, IgA, IgM concentration Quality of life
Qian 2006[22]	Parallel design "Randomly allocated patients" mentioned but no description about randomization procedure No blinding	Total of 70 advanced esophageal cancer patients included 38 assigned to the TCM group and 32 to the control group "Baseline similar" was mentioned	Radiochemotherapy given to two groups From the second week of radiotherapy, TCM decoction given to group A patients until radiotherapy completed Contents of TCM decoction modified according to different TCM signs	Acute esophageal toxic reaction

Abbreviations: DDP, diamminedichloroplatinum (cisplatin); 5-FU, 5-fluorouracil.

−14.67; 95% CI, −17.08–12.26) by giving a self-prepared Huangqi Zengmian decoction compared with chemotherapy only. It resulted in decreasing the rate of CD4/CD8 (MD = 0.16; 95% CI, 0.02–0.30), suggesting improved cellular immune function. Another study[16] reported that CD3 and CD4 concentrations were increased in the TCM group and decreased in the chemotherapy group. The comparison appeared to be statistically significant (MD = 23.60; 95% CI, 21.41–25.79 and MD = 8.00; 95% CI, 5.82–10.18, respectively). In contrast, CD8 concentrations decreased in the TCM group and increased in the chemotherapy group. The difference was statistically significant (MD = −4.70; 95% CI, −6.43–2.97). Furthermore, when comparing the CD4/CD8 levels in the TCM group with those in the chemotherapy group, there was a statistically significant difference (MD = 0.40; 95% CI, 0.33–0.47). Integrated treatment of TCM with chemotherapy versus chemotherapy alone appeared to provide the same effects. CD3 and CD4 concentrations increased significantly in the TCM with chemotherapy group and decreased in the chemotherapy alone group (MD = 23.60; 95% CI, 21.41–25.79 and MD = 8.00, 95% CI, 5.82–10.18, respectively). In addition, CD8 concentrations were decreased in the TCM with chemotherapy group and increased in the chemotherapy group. The difference appeared to be statistically significant (MD = −4.40; 95% CI, −5.89–2.91). There was also a statistically significant difference in CD4/CD8 when comparing TCM plus chemotherapy with chemotherapy alone (MD = 0.60; 95% CI, 0.52–0.68). These results show that TCM treatment alone or in combination with chemotherapy provided improved cellular immune function.

Adverse events
None of the studies reported adverse events resulting from taking TCM. The results can be seen in **Figs. 2 to 5**.

DISCUSSION

Large numbers (possibly thousands) of published articles have assessed TCM in the treatment of esophageal cancer, with almost all of these coming from China. In general, the use of TCM focuses on extending the survival of esophageal cancer patients,[1,2] reducing the adverse reactions of chemo- and radiotherapy,[3] improving the immune system,[4] and providing antitumor processes. As a holistic medical system, TCM treatment is based on the special theory of adjusting the "Ying-Yang" balance to strengthen and support the body's systems.

Some studies[16,19] have shown a survival benefit using integrated TCM with radio- or chemotherapy when compared with radio- or chemotherapy or TCM alone after 5 years. Moreover, other studies[16,22] have found a lower incidence of relapse and cancer metastasis when using radio- or chemotherapy plus TCM when compared with radio- or chemotherapy alone. These results may be due to an improvement in the holistic function of the esophageal cancer patient. For example, three studies[16,20,21] demonstrated the improvement of cellular immune function. Reducing the adverse reactions of radio- and chemotherapy, as reported in three studies,[16,20,22] is also a way of improving the body's power and quality of life.

A total of 119 studies were excluded because they failed to mention "randomly allocated patients," and it was determined that trial staff generally misunderstood the concept of randomization. Some of the studies allocated the patients according to the patients' or trial staffs' opinion, and some were actually retrospective analyses of case records. Although five studies were included, due to an inability to communicate with the authors to confirm the randomization methods and quality issues, none

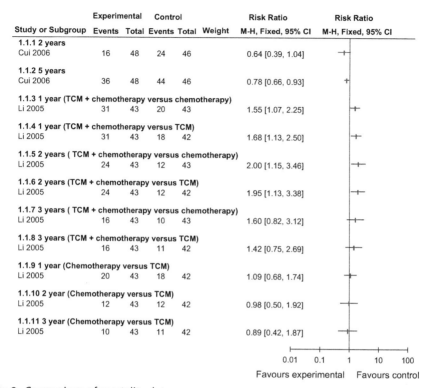

Fig. 2. Comparison of mortality data.

of them was identified as an authentic randomized controlled trial; therefore, the evidence of effects from the included studies of this review is very weak.

There were some potential risks of bias in the included studies that may influence the validity of the results.

High Risk of Selection Bias

Like most of the excluded studies, the five included studies mentioned "randomly allo- cated patients," but the lack of description of the randomization methods meant that some of them were most likely nonrandomized controlled trials.

None of the included studies mentioned how to conceal the allocation procedure and the sequence. From the description, it may be determined that allocation and concealment were not used.

High Risk of Detection Bias

Because blinding was not possible for the oral administration of TCM decoction, the reporting of results, except for mortality data, may be biased. For example, the assessment of quality of life was performed by authors who were not blinded to the trial conditions, which may lead to the increased potential for false-positive results. Valuable assessment about quality of life in a randomized controlled trial should be participant based and should include the use of a validated multidimensional ques- tionnaire completed by the participant with an internationally evaluated minimum stan- dard checklist.[23–25]

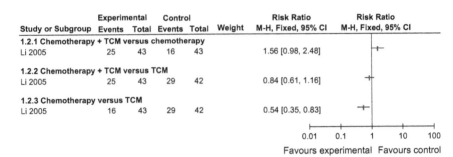

Fig. 3. Comparison of improvement of quality of life.

There is obviously variation in the components of the herbal medical preparations, and each is unique to Chinese traditional herbal medicine. This variation between formulations and batches of treatments is an inevitable consequence of the nature of Chinese traditional medicine. This variation may be a factor that contributes to any heterogeneity between the results of different studies.[26]

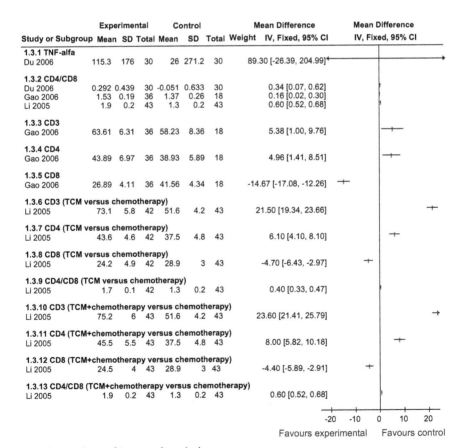

Fig. 4. Comparison of immunology indexes.

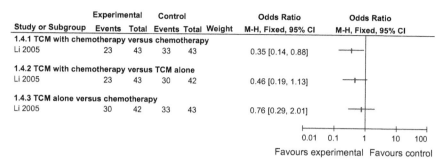

Fig. 5. Comparison of relapse or metastasis of cancer.

A common limitation is that all of the included studies used a self-prepared herbal formulation; therefore, there was high risk of conflict of interest in these studies. The studies using self-prepared herbal formulations provide some evidence of the efficacy of TCM and should encourage further studies by independent researchers from all around the world. These studies will require an improved study design and should include randomization of treatment options.

SUMMARY

Current studies provide some evidence that TCM combined with radio- or chemo-therapy is superior to radio- or chemotherapy alone. Due to methodological issues, there is high risk of bias in these studies. Despite these limitations, we believe that integrated treatment of TCM with radio- or chemotherapy may benefit some esophageal cancer populations. Future well-designed high quality trials are urgently required, and collaborations between Chinese and Western researchers should be strongly encouraged to assist in the development of TCM for esophageal cancer patients.

ACKNOWLEDGMENTS

The authors thank Janet Lilleyman, Iris Gordon, and Cathy Bennett of the Cochrane UGPD Group for advice on writing this review. They also thank all of the authors of the original articles for their patient discussion with Dr. Taixiang Wu and for providing true information from their studies.

REFERENCES

1. Nishihira T, Hashimoto Y, et al. Molecular and cellular features of esophageal cancer cells. J Cancer Res Clin Oncol 1993;119(8):441–9.
2. Pera M. Recent changes in the epidemiology of esophageal cancer. Surg Oncol 2001;10(3):81–90.
3. Blot WJ, Devesa SS, Fraumeni JF Jr. Continuing climb in rates of esophageal adenocarcinoma: an update. JAMA 1993;270(11):1320.
4. Kirby TJ, Rice TW. The epidemiology of esophageal carcinoma: the changing face of a disease. Chest Surg Clin N Am 1994;4(2):217–25.
5. Clark GW, Peters JH, Ireland AP, et al. Nodal metastasis and sites of recurrence after en bloc esophagectomy of adenocarcinoma. Ann Thorac Surg 1994;58(3): 646–54.
6. Steup WH, DeLeyn P, Deneffe I, et al. Tumors of the esophagogastric junction: long-term survival in relation to the pattern of lymph node metastasis and a critical

analysis of the accuracy or inaccuracy of pTNM classification. J Thorac Cardiovasc Surg 1996;111(1):85–94 [discussion: 94–5].

7. Cooper JS, Guo MD, Herskovic A. Chemoradiotherapy of locally advanced esophageal cancer: long-term follow-up of a prospective randomized trial. JAMA 1999;281(17):1623–7.

8. Herskovic A, Martz K, al-Sarraf M. Combined chemotherapy and radiotherapy compared with radiotherapy alone in patients with cancer of the esophagus. N Engl J Med 1992;326(24):1593–8.

9. Chen HH, Zhou HJ, Fang X. Inhibition of human cancer cell line growth and human umbilical vein endothelial cell angiogenesis by artemisinin derivatives in vitro. Pharm Res 2003;48(3):231–6.

10. Wang BS, Liu XF. Clinical observation on effect of Yiqi Huoxue decoction in comprehensive treatment on advanced esophageal cancer. Chin J Integrated Tradit West Med 1999;19(10):589–91.

11. Wei X, Chen ZY, Yang XY, et al. Medicinal herbs for esophageal cancer. Cochrane Database Syst Rev 2007;(2):CD004520.

12. Miller AB, Hoogstraten B, Staquet M, et al. Reporting results of cancer treatment. Cancer 1981;47(1):207–14.

13. Taixiang Wu, Guanjian Liu. The concepts, design, practice and report of allocation concealment and blinding. Chinese Journal of Evidence-Based Medicine 2007;7(3):203–7.

14. Zhao JX, Li XF, Wang XX. Effects of body-resistance strengthening and tumor-suppressing granules on immune adhesion function of red blood cells and expression of metastasis protein CD44 in tumor cells of patients with esophageal carcinoma. World J Gastroenterol 2007;13(32):4360–4.

15. Ren GG, Guo ZX, Zhuang X, et al. A clinical study of traditional Chinese medicine in the treatment of early gastrointestinal dysfunction after vagotomy for esophageal patients. Journal of Sichuan of Traditional Chinese Medicine 2007;25(12):57–8.

16. Li R, Lu P, Kou XG, et al. Effect of the intervention of traditional Chinese medicine on the survival time and quality of life in postoperative esophageal cancer patients. Chin J Clin Rehabil 2005;9(42):63–5.

17. Lu P, Li R, Liang QD, et al. Influence of traditional Chinese medicine on quality of life and function of immune in post-esophagectomy patients with esophageal carcinoma. Journal of Xinxiang Medical College 2006;23(2):121–2.

18. Lu P, Liang QD, Li R, et al. Effect of traditional Chinese medicine on survival and quality of life in patients with esophageal carcinoma after esophagectomy. Chin J Integr Med 2006;12(3):175–9.

19. Cui Q, Jin CJ, Li L, et al. Clinical observation for integrated traditional Chinese and Western medicine in the post-operation patients of esophageal cancer. Modern Journal of Integrated Traditional Chinese and Western Medicine 2006; 15(3):307–8.

20. Du YQ, Li YX, Zhang JR, et al. A clinical study of modified Liu Wei Di Huang Tang with radiotherapy in the treatment of esophageal. Chinese Journal of Cancer Prevention and Treatment 2006;13(18):1428–9.

21. Gao FL, Du HZ. Influence on immune function of Huangqi Zeng Mian Shan decoction in the treatment of perinatal-operation patients with esophageal. Shandong Medicine 2006;46(22):70–1.

22. Qian HY, Zhang P, Huang Y, et al. Traditional Chinese medicine preventing and treatment of esophagitis caused by concurrent radio- and chemotherapy of patients with advanced esophageal cancer. Traditional Chinese Medicinal Materials 2006;29(10):1125–6.

23. Efficace F, Bottomley A, Osoba D, et al. Beyond the development of health-related quality-of-life (HRQOL) measures: a checklist for evaluating HRQOL outcomes in cancer clinical trials. Does HRQOL evaluation in prostate cancer research inform clinical decision making? J Clin Oncol 2003;21(18):3502–11.
24. Efficace F, Horneber M, Lejeune S, et al. Methodological quality of patient-reported outcome research was low in complementary and alternative medicine in oncology. J Clin Epidemiol 2006;59(12):1257–65.
25. Efficace F, Osoba D, Gotay C, et al. Has the quality of health-related quality of life reporting in cancer clinical trials improved over time? Towards bridging the gap with clinical decision making. Ann Oncol 2007;18(4):775–81.
26. Bian ZX, David M, Li YP, et al. Precise reporting of traditional Chinese medicine interventions in randomized controlled trials. Chin J Integr Med 2008;6(7):661–7.

Esophagectomy for the Treatment of Esophageal Cancer

Sandra Tomaszek, MD, Stephen D. Cassivi, MD, MSc*

KEYWORDS

- Esophageal cancer • Esophagectomy • Quality of life
- Postoperative care • Surgical technique

Esophageal cancer remains an uncommon disease in the United States with an incidence rate of 4.6 per 100,000 men and women per year.[1] According to the Surveillance Epidemiology and End Results (SEER) data, an estimated 16,470 men and women were expected to be diagnosed with and 14,280 men and women were expected to die of esophageal cancer in the United States in 2008.[1] The incidence of esophageal adenocarcinoma is increasing faster than any other malignancy in the United States.[2] Esophageal cancer is an aggressive disease with an overall poor prognosis. According to data of the National Cancer Institute, of those with available staging, just over a quarter of esophageal cancer cases are diagnosed at a localized stage, while slightly over a third have locally advanced disease manifested by metastatic spread to regional lymph nodes. Equally just over a third of cases are diagnosed with distant metastases.[1] The corresponding 5-year relative survival rates were: 34.4% for localized esophageal cancer, 17.1% for locally advanced stages and 2.8% for metastatic disease.[1] Surgical resection remains the most definitive form of treatment whether performed alone or in combination with chemotherapy and radiation therapy as part of a multimodality treatment strategy.[3]

PREOPERATIVE PATIENT ASSESSMENT AND STAGING

Esophagogastroduodenoscopy (EGD) commonly is performed as the first diagnostic tool to visualize the extent of the suspected tumor and to obtain biopsies for histologic confirmation of the diagnosis.[4] EGD often is coupled with endoscopic ultrasound (EUS), which is now an essential step in staging esophageal cancer. EUS is the most accurate method of preoperatively assessing T status and has become a standard of care in staging esophageal cancer.[5] EUS also can assess regional lymph nodes and guide endoscopic fine needle aspiration of suspicious lymph nodes.[6,7] CT alone is not very accurate for establishing the nodal status; however, it is an important tool

Division of General Thoracic Surgery, Mayo Clinic, 200 First Street Southwest, Rochester, MN 55905, USA
* Corresponding author.
E-mail address: cassivi.stephen@mayo.edu (S.D. Cassivi).

Gastroenterol Clin N Am 38 (2009) 169–181
doi:10.1016/j.gtc.2009.01.010
0889-8553/09/$ – see front matter © 2009 Elsevier Inc. All rights reserved.

gastro.theclinics.com

of preoperative planning, as it shows potential tumor invasion into adjacent structures.[8] Positron emission tomography (PET) in combination with CT, otherwise known as PET-CT, is useful in searching for distant metastases.[9,10] Finally, if involvement of the trachea by the tumor is suspected, a bronchoscopy should be performed.

Following the staging workup, treatment options should be discussed by the multidisciplinary team and reviewed with the patient. In patients who have early stage disease and without comorbid disease that would contraindicate esophagectomy, surgical resection should be offered as a potentially curative procedure.[11] If patients have locally advanced disease, neoadjuvant chemotherapy and radiation therapy should be considered before proceeding with surgical resection.[8] Proper preoperative assessment of the extent of tumor involvement is very important, as complete resection is a strong prognostic factor on outcome.[12,13] When complete resection (R0) is not possible, no substantial long-term survival can be expected.[14–16]

SURGICAL TECHNIQUES

Various surgical approaches have evolved for esophageal resection. These vary by type, number, and location of incision(s) as well as by choice of conduit used for esophageal replacement and the location and nature of the anastomosis used. Which approach ultimately is employed depends on several factors related to the patient, the tumor, and the surgeon. The patient's past medical and surgical history and their overall functional status will favor one approach over another. The description of each of these varied techniques follows, along with a discussion of the indications, advantages, and disadvantages of each respective approach.

PREOPERATIVE ENDOSCOPY

Before any planned esophageal resection, regardless of the approach, a preoperative endoscopic evaluation of the esophagus, stomach, and proximal duodenum is essential to make a final determination of tumor location, dimension, and extent. It additionally provides the opportunity to assess the suitability of the stomach as a conduit. This can be done as a separate preoperative procedure in the endoscopy suite, requiring usually only moderate sedation, or as a combined procedure, under general anesthetic, just before commencing the formal esophageal resection.

TRANSTHORACIC ESOPHAGECTOMY (IVOR LEWIS ESOPHAGECTOMY)

The original procedure as described by Ivor Lewis in 1946 to treat squamous cell carcinoma of the midesophagus was a two-stage approach including an abdominal incision to mobilize the gastric conduit followed, after an interval of 1 to 2 weeks, by a right thoracotomy for resection and reconstruction of the esophagus.[17] Currently, the transthoracic esophagectomy is performed as a combined procedure requiring only one general anesthetic administration. This remains a favored approach for midesophageal malignancies and is used commonly for distal esophageal carcinomas.[18]

With the patient in the supine position, a midline laparotomy incision is made, and the abdominal cavity is explored to rule out metastatic disease that would preclude a curative procedure and obviate the benefit of proceeding with the operation. Thereafter the stomach is mobilized on the right gastroepiploic artery pedicle. The short gastric vessels are divided, and the lesser sack is entered. The left gastric vessels are dissected out and divided at their origin, while the left gastric and celiac axis lymph nodes (levels 18 and 20, respectively) are removed. Gastric mobility is enhanced by mobilizing the duodenum using the Kocher maneuver. A pyloromyotomy or pyloroplasty is performed to assist with gastric drainage postoperatively. The start of lower esophagus dissection can be accomplished by means of the hiatus to begin this part of the resection that will be completed during the transthoracic portion of the procedure. The abdominal incision then is closed.

The patient is repositioned in the left lateral decubitus position in preparation for a standard right posterolateral thoracotomy, preferably in the fourth interspace (over the top of the fifth rib). After dividing the azygous vein, the esophagus is resected from the apex of the chest down to the hiatus. Paraesophageal and mediastinal lymph nodes are removed en bloc with the esophageal specimen. The stomach then is delivered into the chest and divided along the lesser curvature, taking the left gastric pedicle and lymph nodes with the resected specimen. The thoracic esophagogastrostomy is performed as cephalad as possible, with the goal being to achieve a level at least above the azygous vein. The thoracotomy then is closed after placing a chest tube to drain the pleural space.

TRANSHIATAL ESOPHAGECTOMY

The transhiatal esophagectomy first was performed successfully by the British surgeon Turner in 1933.[19] The concept of esophageal resection without a thoracotomy, however, originally was described by the German anatomist, Denk, in 1913.[20] It was not until it was reintroduced by Orringer in the late 1970s that this operation regained common usage.[21,22] The approach has become popular for treating lower esophageal tumors and early stage lesions such as Barrett's esophagus with high-grade dysplasia.

The surgical procedure as performed routinely consists of an upper midline abdominal incision and left cervical incision. Similar to the transthoracic esophagectomy, the peritoneal cavity initially is explored to rule out metastatic disease. The gastric conduit is mobilized similarly on the right gastroepiploic pedicle.

The esophageal resection is begun by taking a rim of hiatus with the resected lower esophagus to ensure adequate radial margins and also provide a larger aperture through which to continue the transhiatal dissection. Retraction of the hiatus can be used to allow visualization of the dissection quite high up into the mediastinum. Nevertheless, the dissection beyond is carried up to the level of the thoracic inlet and is performed bluntly without direct visualization.

At this point, a left neck incision is performed to allow access to the cervical esophagus. Once the cervical dissection has met the transhiatal dissection, the proximal resection of the esophagus can be performed, usually 1 to 2 cm above the level of the clavicle. The esophagus then is delivered into the abdomen, and a distal resection margin is created on the stomach as described previously with the transthoracic approach. The gastric conduit then is delivered up to the cervical incision by means of the dissected transhiatal route. In this regard, it is important to minimize trauma to the gastric conduit and prevent it from rotating while delivering it through the posterior mediastinum. One frequently applied approach is to place the gastric conduit within a plastic bag that then pulls the stomach up to the neck using a combination of friction and suction to avoid undue damage to the conduit.[23] The cervical esophagogastrostomy then can be performed before closing the neck and abdominal incisions.

TRI-INCISIONAL ESOPHAGECTOMY (MCKEOWN ESOPHAGECTOMY)

The tri-incisional approach for esophagectomy first was described by McKeown[24] in 1976, and consists of a right thoracotomy accompanied by cervical and abdominal incisions. It is an approach employed for both mid- and lower esophageal tumors. It is favored by those surgeons who seek direct visualization of the esophagus during its resection but also prefer a cervical anastomosis.

The initial portion of this procedure is performed through a right posterolateral thoracotomy via the fourth or fifth interspace. The esophagus is dissected as with the transthoracic approach. Once the esophagus and periesophageal tissue and lymph nodes have been mobilized, the chest is closed, and the patient is repositioned in the supine position. The remaining aspects of this operation are completed as described for the transhiatal approach. The laparotomy provides access to mobilize the gastric conduit, which is delivered to the cervical incision by means of the esophageal bed once the esophagus has been resected completely.

The advantages and disadvantages of the tri-incisional esophagectomy are similar to those stated for the transthoracic esophagectomy. In terms of advantages, these include direct visualization of mediastinal structures and mobilization of the thoracic esophagus, which is thought to allow for more complete lymph node dissection.

MINIMALLY INVASIVE ESOPHAGECTOMY

With the aim of reducing the surgical trauma and morbidity typically associated with conventional open esophagectomy, laparoscopic esophagectomy was introduced in the mid-1990s.[25,26] The feasibility of this approach and the ability to reduce postoperative pain and decrease ICU stay and length of hospitalization have been demonstrated in various single-institution studies.[27,28] Nevertheless, the requirement for advanced laparoscopic and thoracoscopic skills has limited the generalized adoption of these types of approaches.[27,29,30]

There are several approaches used to accomplish a minimally invasive esophagectomy.[31] At the authors' institution, the following general approach to the minimally invasive esophagectomy has been adopted. The patient is positioned in the semilithotomy position as for other laparoscopic foregut procedures such as the more commonly performed laparoscopic Nissen fundoplication. The initial laparoscopic access allows for an exploration of the peritoneal cavity to exclude metastases that would obviate the benefit of an esophageal resection. Two 5 mm ports are placed below the costal margins on each side, and two further ports with larger diameter are positioned on the right and left sides of the epigastrium. The laparoscopic preparation of the gastric conduit is accomplished according to the previously described open techniques. Following completion of this, the laparoscopic ports are removed, and the patient is repositioned in a left lateral decubitus position in preparation for a right posterolateral thoracotomy. A 10 mm camera port is inserted at the eighth intercostal space in the midaxillary line. A utility incision is made in the fifth intercostal space between the pectoralis major and latissimus dorsi muscles. A 10 mm working port is placed posterior to the scapula at the fifth intercostal space. A second 10 mm working port is placed at the eighth intercostal space posteriorly. Through these ports, the azygous vein first is divided allowing the esophagus to be visualized and dissected along its entire length along with its associated lymph node tissue. Once the esophagus is dissected entirely, the stomach can be brought up into the chest through the hiatus. It is essential to preserve the correct orientation of the stomach while bringing it up into the chest to avoid ischemia or obstruction of the conduit. The resected esophagus and portion of proximal stomach are removed through the utility port within a surgical bag to avoid port site contamination. The esophagogastrostomy anastomosis then can be completed thoracoscopically.

The main controversy regarding the minimally invasive approaches to esophagectomy relates to whether these approaches achieve an equivalent oncologic result. Randomized, prospective trials comparing conventional open techniques with minimally invasive approaches have not been done. The likelihood of these being completed is also in question. Nevertheless, nonrandomized trials have shown that minimally invasive approaches are safe and comparable to the open approaches with regard to postoperative recovery and short-term survival.[30–33] These also have shown that the duration of the minimally invasive esophagectomy is usually significantly longer than the conventional open approach.[32] Because of the relative novelty of these techniques and therefore lack of long-term follow-up, there are insufficient data to determine long-term survival, the key question for proof of oncologic adequacy.

COMPARISON OF SURGICAL APPROACHES

When comparing the different surgical approaches for esophagectomy, the various procedures provide options that allow for individualizing the operation to the patient and the specifics of their tumor. Midesophageal cancers, especially larger or more bulky tumors, tend to be better approached by direct visualization by means of a transthoracic or tri-incisional approach. The transhiatal or minimally invasive approaches may be favored in situations where the patient may have undue respiratory compromise from a thoracotomy required by the transthoracic or tri-incisional esophagectomies.

Whereas the cervical anastomosis of the transhiatal and tri-incisional approaches is associated with less postoperative reflux complications, it is associated with higher rates of anastomotic leaks than the transthoracic esophagectomy with an intrathoracic anastomosis. Conversely, a cervical anastomotic leak generally is tolerated better and easier to manage than the much more morbid intrathoracic anastomotic leak.[22]

Comparative studies of transhiatal and transthoracic esophagectomies show no significant difference in the overall morbidity and mortality of both approaches and equivalent long-term survival.[34–37] It is therefore a matter for the surgeon to decide on the best approach to esophageal resection for each patient depending on his or her specific condition and nature of the malignancy. A surgeon who is adept at all of these approaches is better able to individualize the surgical procedure to best fit the particular needs of the patient.

OPTIONS FOR ESOPHAGEAL REPLACEMENT CONDUIT

There are several options for conduits to replace the resected esophagus. The most commonly employed conduit is the stomach, while other options include pedicled segments of colon or jejunum and the infrequently used small bowel free graft.[38] The advantage of the stomach as a conduit relates to its more constant and reliable blood supply, its relatively easier dissection and preparation, and the need for only one anastomosis.[39] Prior gastric surgery, including prior fundoplication, may preclude the successful use of the stomach as a replacement conduit.[40] Similarly, a poorly placed gastrostomy may risk rendering the gastric conduit unusable for esophageal replacement.[41] Finally, in the case of Siewert type 3 tumors, emanating from below the gastroesophageal junction, total gastrectomy with distal esophagectomy appears to be the best option. Reconstruction usually is accomplished using a roux-en-y esophagojejunostomy.[42]

If reconstruction with a gastric conduit is not possible, replacement with either colon or jejunum is considered. The first reports about the use of colon as a replacement graft after esophageal resection were published in 1911.[43,44] Advantages of the colon conduit are a relatively consistent vascular anatomy, resistance to gastro–biliary reflux, intrinsic peristalsis, and the ability to maintain the stomach in the abdomen as a reservoir.[45] Reconstruction of the esophagus with colonic interposition often is adopted for cases of congenital esophageal atresia but only occasionally as a conduit after esophagectomy for carcinoma.[46] Patients should undergo a thorough preoperative assessment including a colonoscopy if a colon interposition is planned.[46] Mesenteric angiography may be indicated to assess blood supply if there are questions of peripheral vascular disease.[46] Colonic interposition is associated with higher rates of mortality and morbidity, including an increased anastomotic leak rate and conduit failure rate.[39,40,46]

Jejunum as an esophageal replacement conduit can be used as either a pedicled graft to replace a short segment of distal esophagus or free graft extending higher toward and into the neck. Free jejunal grafts are not the conduit of first choice. They rarely are used and usually only for salvage situations when primary reconstruction with stomach or colon has failed.[40] The advantages of the jejunal conduit are the avoidance of preoperative bowel preparation, active intrinsic peristalsis, and typically good luminal size match between the jejunum and esophagus.[45]

POSTOPERATIVE MANAGEMENT

At the time of the operation, a nasogastric tube usually is placed to decompress the stomach during the first 1 to 2 days after surgery. This is in addition to the commonly performed pyloromyotomy or pyloroplasty to promote antegrade drainage of gastric contents.[47,48] Gastric emptying also can be assisted with the postoperative use of prokinetic agents such as erythromycin or metoclopramide.[49] In a further effort to avoid gastric distention in the early postoperative period, many thoracic surgeons discourage any oral intake for the first 4 to 6 weeks while using the feeding jejunostomy to provide nutrition in the interim.[39]

One of the potential major complications of esophagectomy is an anastomotic leak. This has been reported in the modern literature to range from 0.8% to over 20%.[50–55] Typically cervical anastomoses have a leak rate between 5% and 15%, while for intrathoracic anastomoses this rate is usually between 1% and 4%.[39] Identifying such anastomotic leaks is the object of much attention in the early postoperative period. Clinical suspicion based on physical findings and basic laboratory investigations is the initial method used for detection. The clinical scenario often will be very obvious in the case of a large anastomotic disruption. Bile exiting by means of the right chest tube following a transthoracic esophagectomy or saliva exuding from the neck incision after a transhiatal esophagectomy are incontrovertible signs requiring no further confirmatory testing. When these clear-cut signs are not present, the diagnostic modality most commonly employed is the contrast swallow.[56,57] A postoperative contrast swallow is used almost routinely to evaluate intrathoracic anastomoses before patients are allowed to resume oral intake, because an intrathoracic leak is usually both more challenging to diagnose and more difficult to treat than one in the neck. Conversely, a radiologic leak, at the cervical level, without associated clinical findings, is usually inconsequential and requires no specific therapeutic intervention. Therefore, postoperative contrast studies have become less of a routine following transhiatal or tri-incisional esophagectomy that employs a cervical anastomosis. The decreased use of contrast studies has been advocated to avoid the real risk of aspiration pneumonia.[58]

POSTOPERATIVE COMPLICATIONS AFTER ESOPHAGECTOMY

Despite continued surgical advances, as noted previously, anastomotic leaks remain a common complication after esophagectomy.[50] Recent modifications using surgical stapling devices have led to decreased leak rates both in cervical and intrathoracic locations.[59,60] Early leaks most frequently present with fulminant clinical deterioration of the patient within the first 72 hours of surgery needing intravenous fluid resuscitation and immediate surgical exploration and repair.[61] Early leaks most likely are caused by graft necrosis or profound technical problems at the anastomotic site.[39,45,62] Smaller leaks become evident later by means of wound drainage, leukocytosis, or other nonspecific clinical symptoms. Treatment often depends on the location and severity of the anastomotic leak. Generally, cervical anastomotic leaks can be managed with appropriate drainage, usually by means of a cervical incision. In contrast, intrathoracic leaks typically have been associated with high mortality rates because of mediastinitis. In the past, these have been managed by reoperation, proximal esophageal diversion, and return at a much later date for reconstitution of the gastrointestinal continuity by means such as a colonic interposition. Recently there have been increasing reports of successful primary repair, suggesting a role for aggressive anastomotic salvage strategies.[63]

Anastomotic strictures are another distinct complication following esophagec-tomy.[61,64] The reported incidence of strictures varies widely from as low as 1%[65] to as high as 50%.[66] Dysphagia is the most common cited complaint, and the incidence is therefore largely dependent on the diligence of eliciting this very subjective symptom during follow-up. Although different than anastomotic leaks, strictures often are associated with prior occurrence of a leak. Most occurrences of these benign strictures appear within the first few months after surgery. Any strictures presenting later should be evaluated specifically to rule out tumor recurrence. When not caused by tumor recurrence, late strictures are most often the result of reflux from the gastric conduit, more commonly with more distally placed anastomoses.[51,67]

Pulmonary complications are frequent after esophagectomy, with rates of 2% up to 20%,[50,51,53,55,68] ranging from aspiration pneumonia, pneumonitis, prolonged require-ment for ventilator support, adult respiratory distress syndrome, and fulminant pulmo-nary sepsis with multiorgan failure.[69] Although some patients are known to have preoperative risk factors such as emphysema, cigarette smoking, and prior radiation including that employed now commonly for neoadjuvant therapy, the true pathophys-iological mechanism of postoperative pulmonary morbidity remains incompletely understood.[69] Recurrent laryngeal nerve injury is a rather seldom complication of 1% to 5%.[50,51,55,68] This injury is associated with considerable morbidity because of associated pulmonary complications resulting from the effects of aspiration.[70]

Thoracic duct injury with subsequent chylothorax is a rare, yet devastating compli-cation after esophagectomy, with reported incidence of around 1%.[50–53,55,68] It pres-ents clinically by increased chest tube outputs of creamy-colored fluid, and it is diagnosed by quantifying the triglyceride level and identifying chylomicrons within the effusion fluid. Conservative treatment, consisting of eliminating gastrointestinal feeding and replacing this with parenteral nutrition, often is attempted initially. If high-volume chest tube outputs persist, however, reoperation with ligation of the supradiaphragmatic thoracic duct is indicated.[71]

QUALITY OF LIFE AND FUNCTIONAL STATUS AFTER ESOPHAGECTOMY

Contemporary evaluations of surgical procedures such as esophagectomy increas-ingly are based not only on measures of morbidity and mortality but also on postoperative functional status and quality of life.[72–77] General and disease-specific instruments exist to measure quality of life following esophagectomy. In 1997, McLarty and colleagues[51] assessed the quality of life of 64 long-term survivors after esophagectomy for stage 1 and 2 esophageal cancer. The Medical Outcomes Study 36-Item Short-Form Health Survey (MOS SF-36) was applied, and findings were compared with the national norm matched for gender and age. Overall quality of life was not impaired; however, physical function scores significantly decreased with a trend toward decreased level of energy. Mental health status on the other hand was superior to the norm. Occurrence of an anastomotic leak had adverse effects on scores, reflecting health perception. Results from the esophageal function questionnaire reported dysphagia to solid and pureed diet, postprandial dumping, and reflux to be common even in long-term survivors. Significantly less reflux symptoms with cervical anastomosis than with intrathoracic anastomosis were observed.[51] Patients who had a cervical anastomosis on the other hand reported having significantly more dumping than those who had an intrathoracic anastomosis.[72]

Disease-specific tools for evaluating quality of life in esophageal cancer have been developed and standardized in the past years. In a prospective study design, the validated European Organization for Research and Treatment of Cancer general quality-of-life-questionnaire (EORTC QLQ-C30) with the esophageal-specific module (QLQ-OES18) have been applied by Lagergren and colleagues[78] before and at least 3 years after esophagectomy for cancer to assess health-related quality of life. Forty-seven of 90 operated patients survived at least 3 years. Most scores recovered to preoperative levels except for physical function, breathlessness, diarrhea, and reflux, which were rated as significantly worse. Similar findings were reported by other investigators.[79] Deterioration of quality of life was not affected by the chosen surgical approach or by the anastomotic site.[80] Another useful quality of life tool is the Functional Assessment of Cancer Therapy-Esophageal (FACT-E), which has been developed and validated as a specific quality-of-life tool for esophageal cancer.[81,82] Overall, long-term survivors of esophagectomy for cancer show transient decreases in certain quality-of-life parameters that seem to rebound back to baseline over time.

LOW- VERSUS HIGH-VOLUME CENTERS

Patients diagnosed with esophageal cancer commonly are referred to a specialized center for further staging and evaluation of treatment options. With esophagectomy being associated with a relatively high operative morbidity and mortality, there has been increasing investigation as to whether volume of cases affects overall outcome. It has been reported that operative mortality from esophagectomy is threefold higher in low-volume centers performing less than two esophagectomies annually as compared with so-called high-volume centers performing more than 19 per year.[83] In a similar study, the mortality risk was over fourfold higher in low-volume centers with four or less cases per year as compared with centers performing 11 or more esophagectomies annually.[84] These volume-to-outcome relationships have been reproduced in various other investigations.[85–87] It is especially noteworthy in this era of increased cost awareness, that high-volume surgeons (more than 11 esophagectomies per year) provide care at significantly lower (10.6%) inpatient costs.[88]

Patients may benefit from referral to high-volume centers, as their multidisciplinary teams are able to provide experienced and skilled patient care, potentially resulting in fewer complications and low mortality rates.[8,22,34,89] Yet, in some studies, high hospital volume in and of itself did not necessarily guarantee superior outcome.[84–86]

SUMMARY

Esophagectomy remains a key therapeutic option in treating patients who have localized esophageal cancer. Tailoring the surgical approach to the patient and the nature of his or her malignancy is essential. Over time, advances in staging, preoperative assessment, operative techniques, and postoperative care have resulted in decreased operative mortality.

REFERENCES

1. National Cancer Institute. Surveillance Epidemiology and End Results (SEER) Web site. Available at: http://seer.cancer.gov/statfacts/html/esoph.html. Accessed August 18, 2008.
2. Pohl H, Welch HG. The role of overdiagnosis and reclassification in the marked increase of esophageal adenocarcinoma incidence. J Natl Cancer Inst 2005; 97:142–6.
3. McKian KP, Miller RC, Cassivi SD, et al. Curing patients with locally advanced esophageal cancer: an update on multimodality therapy. Dis Esophagus 2006; 19:448–53.
4. Moretó M. Diagnosis of esophagogastric tumors. Endoscopy 2005;37:26–32.
5. Rice TW. Clinical staging of esophageal carcinoma. CT, EUS, and PET. Chest Surg Clin N Am 2000;10:471–85.
6. Vázques-Sequeiros E, Wiersema MJ, Clain JE, et al. Impact of lymph node staging on therapy of esophageal carcinoma. Gastroenterology 2003;125: 1626–35.
7. Gines A, Cassivi SD, Martenson JA Jr, et al. Impact of endoscopic ultrasonography and physician specialty on the management of patients with esophagus cancer. Dis Esophagus 2008;21:241–50.
8. Pennathur A, Luketich JD. Resection for esophageal cancer: strategies for optimal management. Ann Thorac Surg 2008;85:S751–6.
9. Koshy M, Esiashvilli N, Landry JC, et al. Multiple management modalities in esophageal cancer: epidemiology, presentation and progression, work-up, and surgical approaches. Oncologist 2004;9:137–46.
10. Choi JY, Jang HJ, Shim YM, et al. 18F-FDG PET in patients with esophageal squamous cell carcinoma undergoing curative surgery: prognostic implications. J Nucl Med 2004;45:1843–50.
11. Luketich JD, Pennathur A. How to keep the treatment of esophageal disease in the surgeon's hands. Ann Thorac Surg 2008;85:S760–3.
12. Greene FL, Page DL, Fleming ID, et al. Esophageal cancer staging. In: AJCC cancer staging manual. 6th edition. New York: Springer-Verlag; 2002. p. 91–8.
13. Barbour AP, Rizk NP, Gonem M, et al. Adenocarcinoma of the gastroesophageal junction: influence of esophageal resection margin and operative approach on outcome. Ann Surg 2007;246:1–8.
14. Dexter SP, Sue-Ling S, McMahon MJ, et al. Circumferential resection margin involvement: an independent predictor of survival following surgery for oesophageal cancer. Gut 2001;48:667–70.
15. Hofstetter W, Swisher SG, Correa AM, et al. Treatment outcomes of resected esophageal cancer. Ann Surg 2002;236:376–84.
16. Kelson DP, Winter KA, Gunderson LL, et al. Long-term results of RTOG Trial 8911 (USA Intergroup 113): a random assignment trial comparison of chemotherapy followed by surgery compared with surgery alone for esophageal cancer. J Clin Oncol 2007;25:3719–25.

17. Lewis I. The surgical treatment of carcinoma of the esophagus with special reference to a new operation for growths of the middle third. Br J Surg 1946;34:18–31.
18. Nichols FC, Allen MS, Deschamps C, et al. Ivor Lewis esophagogastrectomy. Surg Clin North Am 2005;85:583–92.
19. Turner GG. Excision of thoracic esophagus for carcinoma with construction of extrathoracic gullet. Lancet 1933;2:1315–6.
20. Denk W. [Zur Radikaloperation des Osophaguskarzinoms]. Zentralbl Chir 1913; 40:1065–8 [German].
21. Orringer MB, Sloan H. Esophagectomy without thoracotomy. J Thorac Cardiovasc Surg 1978;76:643–54.
22. Orringer MB, Marshall B, Chang AC, et al. Two thousand transhiatal esophagectomies: changing trends, lessons learned. Ann Surg 2007;246:363–74.
23. Inculet RI, Finley RJ, Cooper JD. A new technique for delivering the stomach or colon to the neck following total esophagectomy. Ann Thorac Surg 1988;45:451–2.
24. McKeown K. Total 3-stage oesophagectomy for cancer of the oesophagus. Br J Surg 1976;63:259–62.
25. DePaula AL, Hashiba K, Ferreira EA, et al. Laparoscopic transhiatal esophagectomy with esophagogastroplasty. Surg Laparosc Endosc 1995;5:1–5.
26. Swanstrom LL, Hansen P. Laparoscopic total esophagectomy. Arch Surg 1997; 132:943–9.
27. Luketich JD, Alvelo-Rivera M, Buenaventura PO, et al. Minimally invasive esophagectomy: outcomes in 222 patients. Ann Surg 2003;238:486–95.
28. Litle VR, Buenaventura PO, Luketich JD. Minimally invasive resection for esophageal cancer. Surg Clin North Am 2002;82:711–28.
29. Kent MS, Schuchert M, Fernando H, et al. Minimally invasive esophagectomy: state of the art. Dis Esophagus 2006;19:137–45.
30. Böttger T, Terzic A, Müller M, et al. Minimally invasive transhiatal and transthoracic esophagectomy. Surg Endosc 2007;21:1695–700.
31. Law S. Minimally invasive techniques for oesophageal cancer surgery. Best Pract Res Clin Gastroenterol 2006;20:925–40.
32. Smithers BM, Gotley DC, Martin I, et al. Comparison of the outcomes between open and minimally invasive esophagectomy. Ann Surg 2007;245:232–40.
33. Pierre AF, Luketich JD. Technique and role of minimally invasive esophagectomy for premalignant and malignant diseases of the esophagus. Surg Oncol Clin N Am 2002;11:337–50.
34. Connors RC, Reuben BC, Neumayer LA, et al. Comparing outcomes after transthoracic and transhiatal esophagectomy: a 5-year prospective cohort of 17,395 patients. J Am Coll Surg 2007;205:735–40.
35. Gluch L, Smith RC, Bambach CP, et al. Comparison of outcomes following transhiatal or Ivor Lewis esophagectomy for esophageal carcinoma. World J Surg 1999;23:271–6.
36. Hulscher JB, van Sandick JW, de Boer AG, et al. Extended transthoracic resection compared with limited transhiatal resection for adenocarcinoma of the esophagus. N Engl J Med 2002;347:1662–9.
37. Chang AC, Ji H, Birkmeyer NJ, et al. Outcomes after transhiatal and transthoracic esophagectomy for cancer. Ann Thorac Surg 2008;85:424–9.
38. Bredenberg CE, Hiebert CA, et al. Selection and placement of conduits. In: Patterson GA, Cooper JD, Deslauriers J, editors. Pearson's thoracic & esophageal surgery. 3rd edition. Philadelphia: Churchill Livingstone Elsevier; 2008. p. 555–62.

39. Cassivi SD. Leaks, strictures, and necrosis: a review of anastomotic complications following esophagectomy. Semin Thorac Cardiovasc Surg 2004;16: 124–32.

40. Mansour KA, Bryan FC, Carlson GW. Bowel interposition for esophageal replacement: twenty-five-year experience. Ann Thorac Surg 1997;64:752–6.

41. Ohnmacht GA, Allen MS, Cassivi SD, et al. Percutaneous endoscopic gastrostomy risks rendering the gastric conduit unusable for esophagectomy. Dis Esophagus 2006;19:311–2.

42. Shen KR, Cassivi SD, Deschamps C, et al. Surgical treatment of tumors of the proximal stomach with involvement of the distal esophagus: a 26-year experience with Siewert type-III tumors. J Thorac Cardiovasc Surg 2006;132:755–62.

43. Kelling G. [Oesophagoplastik mit Hilfe des Querkolon]. Zentralbl Chir 1911;38: 1209–12 [German].

44. Vulliet H. [De l'oesophagoplastie et des diverses modifications]. Sem Med 1911; 31:529–34 [French].

45. Wormuth JK, Heitmiller RF. Esophageal conduit necrosis. Thorac Surg Clin 2006; 16:11–22.

46. Cerfolio RJ, Allen MS, Deschamps C, et al. Esophageal replacement by colon interposition. Ann Thorac Surg 1995;59:1382–4.

47. Law S, Cheung MC, Fok M, et al. Pyloroplasty and pyloromyotomy in gastric replacement of the esophagus after esophagectomy: a randomized controlled trial. J Am Coll Surg 1997;184:630–6.

48. Urschel JD, Blewett CJ, Young JE, et al. Pyloric drainage (pyloroplasty) or no drainage in gastric reconstruction after esophagectomy: a meta-analysis of randomized controlled trials. Dig Surg 2002;19:160–4.

49. Burt M, Scott A, Williard WC, et al. Erythromycin stimulates gastric emptying after esophagectomy with gastric replacement: a randomized clinical trial. J Thorac Cardiovasc Surg 1996;111:649–54.

50. Orringer MB, Marshall B, Iannettoni MD. Transhiatal esophagectomy: clinical experience and refinements. Ann Surg 1999;230:392–400.

51. McLarty AJ, Deschamps C, Trastek VF, et al. Esophageal resection for cancer of the esophagus: long-term function and quality of life. Ann Thorac Surg 1997;63:1568–72.

52. Gockel I, Exner C, Junginger T. Morbidity and mortality after esophagectomy for esophageal carcinoma: a risk analysis. World J Surg Oncol 2005;3:37.

53. King RM, Pairolero PC, Trastek VF, et al. Ivor Lewis esophagogastrectomy for carcinoma of the esophagus: early and late functional results. Ann Thorac Surg 1987;44:119–22.

54. Braghetto I, Csendes A, Cardemil G, et al. Open transthoracic or transhiatal esophagectomy versus minimally invasive esophagectomy in terms of morbidity, mortality and survival. Surg Endosc 2006;20:1681–6.

55. Atkins BZ, Shah AS, Hutcheson KA, et al. Reducing hospital morbidity and mortality following esophagectomy. Ann Thorac Surg 2004;78:1170–6.

56. Bruce J, Krukowski ZH, Al-Khairy G, et al. Systematic review of the definition and measurement of anastomotic leak after gastrointestinal surgery. Br J Surg 2001; 88:1157–68.

57. Griffin SM, Lamb PJ, Dresner SM, et al. Diagnosis and management of a mediastinal leak following radical oesophagectomy. Br J Surg 2001;88:1346–51.

58. Tirnaksiz MB, Deschamps C, Allen MS, et al. Effectiveness of screening aqueous contrast swallow in detecting clinically significant anastomotic leaks after esophagectomy. Eur Surg Res 2007;37:123–8.

59. Behzadi A, Nichols FC, Cassivi SD, et al. Esophagogastrectomy: the influence of stapled versus hand-sewn anastomosis on outcome. J Gastrointest Surg 2005;9: 1031–42.
60. Orringer MB, Marshall B, Iannettoni MD. Eliminating the cervical esophagogastric anastomotic leak with a side-to-side stapled anastomosis. J Thorac Cardiovasc Surg 2000;119:277–88.
61. Mitchell JD. Anastomotic leak after esophagectomy. Thorac Surg Clin 2006;16:1–9.
62. Page RD, Shackcloth MJ, Russell GN, et al. Surgical treatment of anastomotic leaks after oesophagectomy. Eur J Cardiothorac Surg 2005;27:337–43.
63. Crestanello JA, Deschamps C, Cassivi SD, et al. Selective management of intra-thoracic anastomotic leak after esophagectomy. J Thorac Cardiovasc Surg 2005; 129:254–60.
64. Rice TW. Anastomotic stricture complicating esophagectomy. Thorac Surg Clin 2006;16:63–73.
65. Huang GJ. Replacement of the esophagus with the stomach. In: Shields TW, editor. General thoracic surgery. 5th edition. Philadelphia: Lippincott Williams & Wilkins; 2000. p. 1723–32.
66. Dewar L, Gelfand G, Finley RJ, et al. Factors affecting cervical anastomotic leak and stricture formation following esophagogastrectomy and gastric tube interposition. Am J Surg 1992;163:484–9.
67. De Leyn P, Coosemans W, Lerut T. Early and late functional results in patients with intrathoracic gastric replacement after oesophagectomy for carcinoma. Eur J Cardiothorac Surg 1992;6:79–85.
68. Visbal AL, Allen MS, Miller DL, et al. Ivor Lewis esophagectomy for esophageal cancer. Ann Thorac Surg 2001;71:1803–8.
69. Atkins BZ, D'Amico TA. Respiratory complications after esophagectomy. Thorac Surg Clin 2006;16:35–48.
70. Wright CD, Zeitels SM. Recurrent laryngeal nerve injuries after esophagectomy. Thorac Surg Clin 2006;16:23–33.
71. Cerfolio RJ. Chylothorax after esophagectomy. Thorac Surg Clin 2006;16:49–52.
72. Deschamps C, Nichols FC, Cassivi SD, et al. Long-term function and quality of life after esophageal resection for cancer and Barrett's. Surg Clin North Am 2005;85:649–56.
73. Fernandez FG, Meyers BF. Quality of life after esophagectomy. Semin Thorac Cardiovasc Surg 2004;16:152–9.
74. Lipscomb J, Donaldson MS, Arora NK, et al. Cancer outcomes research. J Natl Cancer Inst Monographs 2004;33:178–97.
75. Beitz J, Gnecco C, Justice R. Quality-of-life end points in cancer clinical trials: the US Food and Drug Administration perspective. J Natl Cancer Inst Monographs 1996;20:7–9.
76. Enzinger PC, Mayer RJ. Esophageal cancer. N Engl J Med 2003;349:2241–52.
77. Wu PC, Posner MC. The role of surgery in the management of oesophageal cancer. Lancet Oncol 2003;4:481–8.
78. Lagergren P, Avery KN, Hughes R, et al. Health-related quality of life among patients cured by surgery for esophageal cancer. Cancer 2007;110:686–93.
79. Djärv T, Lagergren J, Blazeby JM, et al. Long-term health-related quality of life following surgery for oesophageal cancer. Br J Surg 2008;95:1121–6.
80. Egberts JH, Schniewind B, Bestmann B, et al. Impact of the site of anastomosis after oncologic esophagectomy on quality of life—a prospective, longitudinal outcome study. Ann Surg Oncol 2008;15:566–75.
81. Darling G, Eton DT, Sulman J, et al. Validation of the functional assessment of cancer therapy esophageal cancer subscale. Cancer 2006;107:854–63.

82. Conroy T, Uwer L, Deblock M. Health-related quality-of-life assessment in gastro-intestinal cancer: are results relevant for clinical practice? Curr Opin Oncol 2007; 19:401–6.

83. Birkmeyer JD, Siewers AE, Finlayson EV, et al. Hospital volume and surgical mortality in the United States. N Engl J Med 2002;346:1128–37.

84. Migliore M, Choong CK, Lim E, et al. A surgeon's case volume of oesophagectomy for cancer strongly influences the operative mortality rate. Eur J Cardiothorac Surg 2007;32:375–80.

85. Verhoef C, Van de Weyer R, Schaapveld M, et al. Better survival in patients with esophageal cancer after surgical treatment in university hospitals: a plea for performance by surgical oncologists. Ann Surg Oncol 2007;14:1678–87.

86. Rouvelas I, Jia C, Viklund P, et al. Surgeon volume and postoperative mortality after oesophagectomy for cancer. Eur J Surg Oncol 2007;33:162–8.

87. Wouters MW, Wijnhoven BP, Karim-Kos HE, et al. High volume versus low volume for esophageal resections for cancer: the essential role of case mix adjustments based on clinical data. Ann Surg Oncol 2008;15:80–7.

88. Ho V, Aloia T. Hospital volume, surgeon volume, and patient costs for cancer surgery. Med Care 2008;46:718–25.

89. Dimick JB, Pronovost PJ, Cowan JA, et al. Surgical volume and quality of care for esophageal resection: do high-volume hospitals have fewer complications? Ann Thorac Surg 2003;75:337–41.

Future Developments in Esophageal Cancer Research

Jaffer A. Ajani, MD

KEYWORDS

- Esophageal cancer • Combine modality therapy • Biomarkers
- Individualization of therapy • Epidemiology

Each year esophageal carcinoma accounts for more than 460,000 new cases and approximately 375,000 deaths worldwide.[1] The incidence has steadily risen in the United States over the past 17 years.[2] Squamous cell histology is more frequent in the endemic areas, whereas adenocarcinoma histology is more frequent in the nonendemic areas. An alarming as well as intriguing aspect is the increase in the incidence of adenocarcinoma in the West and the shift in the location to the lower third of the esophagus and gastroesophageal junction.[3,4] Although Scotland and England have the highest incidence of adenocarcinoma of the esophagus in the world, there are no definite clues as to why.[5] Squamous cell carcinoma has been associated with smoking and alcohol, whereas adenocarcinoma is associated with obesity, gastroesophageal reflux disease, and Barrett's metaplasia.[6] Whereas previously the diagnosis of adenocarcinoma has often been made in executive-type Caucasian men in their late 50s and early 60s, there is now a rise in the incidence of adenocarcinoma in Caucasian women[5] and blacks.[3] It would appear that adenocarcinoma of the esophagus is not a gender- or ethnicity-specific disease but predominantly related to lifestyle factors and that susceptibility has a major role.

Because early detection strategies for esophageal cancer have rarely been implemented, it is commonly diagnosed in an advanced stage resulting in an increasing number of deaths.[4] It is hoped that heightened awareness of the consequences of Barrett's metaplasia might lead to a higher fraction of individuals undergoing surveillance and early detection of adenocarcinoma. A parallel strategy would be to identify individuals who are at high risk for developing adenocarcinoma through molecular epidemiologic studies. Molecular studies hold considerable promise. Various genetic polymorphisms have already been correlated with an increased risk of

Work for this article was supported in part by grants from the UT M. D. Anderson Cancer Center, NCI (CA127672), the Dallas, Park, Cantu, and Smith families, and the River Creek Foundation.

Department of GI Medical Oncology, The University of Texas M. D. Anderson Cancer Center, 1515 Holcombe Boulevard, Unit 426, Houston, TX 77030, USA

E-mail address: jajani@mdanderson.org

Gastroenterol Clin N Am 38 (2009) 183–188
doi:10.1016/j.gtc.2009.01.001

adenocarcinoma of the esophagus, and such findings (when mature) may facilitate targeted surveillance.[7–9] Much work remains to be done to develop a validated risk model. With the advent of emerging technology and a greater understanding of genetic and epigenetic changes in cancer and patient genetics, we will have a better understanding of the reasons why some individuals have a higher risk and why inherent heterogeneity occurs in the clinical biology of esophageal cancer that is commonly encountered.[10–13]

Localized carcinoma of the esophagus is a potentially curable condition, but to provide optimum and effective care it is necessary to establish an experienced infrastructure that exercises a multidisciplinary approach. A multidisciplinary approach requires accurate staging and review of medical data by all involved disciplines (gastroenterology, radiology, medical oncology, surgery, radiation oncology, pathology, and nutrition) before rendering any therapy. Newer techniques to stage cancer have facilitated better patient selection for complex approaches. Among the many new techniques to accurately stage cancer, endoscopic ultrasonography (with an ability to perform fine-needle aspiration of suspected nodes) and positron emission tomography (PET) represent advancements. Changes in serial PET are of particular importance because PET not only provides staging information but also characterizes the clinical biology of esophageal cancer undergoing therapy.[14–20] The future of cancer imaging lies in using more sophisticated technology with new (and specific) imaging targets.[21]

The major source of frustration for patients, their relatives, and the medical team has been the selection of therapy that is likely to be effective and the avoidance of ineffective ones. There is some clarity for early stage cancer. For example, a consensus is emerging for endoscopic mucosal resection as the preferred therapy for patients with T1a cancers and for surgery for those with T1b cancers. There is lack of convincing data when dealing with cancers that are stage II or III; however, in the West, for the commonly diagnosed stages of localized esophageal adenocarcinoma (II or III), preoperative therapy has become increasingly popular[22,23] despite the lack of convincing data in randomized trials.[24–27] One tradition has been to group patients in a certain stage category (eg, combining all patients with stages II and III) and offer everyone the same therapeutic approach. Some patients are cured by this strategy but many are not, and some do not benefit at all. Clearly, all patients sustain considerable toxicities from chemoradiation[28] and complications from surgery.[29] Unfortunately, clinical parameters are not helpful in selecting therapy for patients with stage II or III cancer.[30] It is increasingly clear that residual cancer found in the resected surgical specimen after preoperative therapy (particularly chemoradiation) is a determinant of the patient's long-term outcome.[30–34] The class of cytotoxic agents or the use of induction chemotherapy also does not seem to influence the pathologic response.[35–37] Fluoropyrimidine should be administered with radiation, but the second cytotoxic agent can be a platinum compound, taxane, or camptothecin. The value of the addition of biologics to chemoradiation is being investigated. We should realize that this is simply an extension of an investigative tradition that promotes empiricism.

When asking the question of what tools could be employed to optimize therapy for patients with esophageal cancer, one should first recognize the three subtypes of esophageal cancer that drive the clinical biology and therefore patient outcomes. These subtypes are based on the degree of chemoradiation resistance inherent in the primary tumor. Each subtype could be treated differently and expected to result in a different patient outcome.

Subtype I includes patients whose tumors are extremely chemoradiation sensitive and in whom no cancer cells are found in the surgical specimen (pathologic complete response). Approximately 25% of patients (irrespective of whether the tumor is clinical stage II or III) achieve a pathologic complete response. Their 5-year survival rate often exceeds 50%.[31,33,34] One could argue that if we could identify these patients before therapy is initiated, observation after chemoradiation would be a strong consideration (ie, an attempt at esophagus preservation with surgery used as salvage). Although some biomarkers are associated with pathologic response, currently these are not well refined, and the specificity is too low for implementation.[38,39]

Subtype II includes patients whose tumors are partially sensitive to chemoradiation. Approximately 1% to 50% have residual cancer found in the surgical specimen.[30] These patients (if identified before any therapy is delivered) seem to benefit from chemoradiation and surgery. They have a moderate lifespan and moderate metastatic potential.[30,40]

Table 1
Future of esophageal cancer research

Area of Research	Future Possibilities	Comments
Epidemiology	Molecular epidemiology will dominate this arena.	To study large cohorts of patients, collaboration among institutions is necessary.
Etiology	Better understanding of specific causes of adenocarcinoma is highly likely.	Knowledge will fuel prevention strategies.
Prevention/early detection	Better understanding of susceptibility factors (genetic or lifestyle related) will arise. Creation of a multifaceted risk model will follow.	Identification of high-risk populations and tailored surveillance are necessary.
Imaging	More specific imaging to identify and guide therapies will be developed.	Biomarkers will have a greater role in complementing imaging advances.
Staging	Improved imaging and other technologies will allow more sophisticated staging that will be able to predict biologic behavior of cancer.	Patients will be subgrouped in a more meaningful manner than is possible today. Metabolic and target-specific imaging will define biology.
Therapy for localized cancer	Individualization of therapy will be possible by studying molecular biology of cancer and patient genetics.	Selection of optimal therapy might become the norm and will reduce cost and morbidity.
Radiotherapy	Further evolution of radiation techniques to reduce normal tissue toxicities is likely.	Sophisticated tumor imaging will have an increasing role in radiation planning for esophageal carcinoma.
Surgery	Minimally invasive surgery will evolve and will be employed in select cases.	Evolving technology might allow image-guided surgery and also identification of involved nodal groups.
Personalized medicine	Integration of clinical and molecular information could lead to validated individualized approaches.	This effort will reduce cost, frustration, morbidity, and uncertainties but at the same time might identify new exploitable therapeutic targets.

Subtype III includes patients whose tumors are extremely resistant to chemoradiation. More than 50% have residual cancer found in the surgical specimen.[30] Clearly, these patients need to be identified as soon as possible (preferably before therapy is initiated, but even early during therapy would be better than what is done today) to avoid chemoradiation and proceed directly to surgery. Their prognosis is very poor.

The progress that has been made against esophageal carcinoma is limited and certainly not impressive. Many relevant issues remain, including whether to deal with squamous cell carcinoma differently than adenocarcinoma, the dose of radiation and the fractionation scheme, how to orchestrate a multidisciplinary approach, the therapy of T4 and M1 cancers, specific surgical techniques, the development of a risk model for surgical therapy and chemoradiation therapy, the frequency of follow-up and with what staging methods after definitive therapy, the programmatic approach to molecular biologic studies, and so on. These issues are beyond the scope of this article. **Table 1** summarizes my thoughts on what the future might hold. Fortunately, the future appears promising. Nevertheless, the startling increase in the incidence of adenocarcinoma suggests that esophageal adenocarcinoma is the disease of future and in 20 years might surpass colon cancer. Although this sounds unlikely, we will see. I hope that the National Institute of Health is paying attention, because it has not yet set aside dedicated funds to study adenocarcinoma of the esophagus or gastroesophageal junction.

REFERENCES

1. Parkin DM, Bray F, Ferlay J, et al. Global cancer statistics, 2002. CA Cancer J Clin 2005;55(2):74–108.
2. American Cancer Society. Cancer statistics. Available at: www.ACS.org. Accessed October 17, 2007.
3. Brown LM, Devesa SS, Chow WH. Incidence of adenocarcinoma of the esophagus among white Americans by sex, stage, and age. J Natl Cancer Inst 2008; 100(16):1184–7.
4. Pohl H, Welch HG. The role of overdiagnosis and reclassification in the marked increase of esophageal adenocarcinoma incidence. J Natl Cancer Inst 2005; 97(2):142–6.
5. Comparison with other European countries. In: Oesophageal (gullet) cancer. London: UK Cancer Research; 2008. Available at: http://info.cancerresearchuk.org/cancerstats/types/oesophagus/incidence/. Accessed November 1, 2008.
6. Brown LM, Swanson CA, Gridley G, et al. Adenocarcinoma of the esophagus: role of obesity and diet. J Natl Cancer Inst 1995;87(2):104–9.
7. Izzo J, Papadimitrakopoulou VA, Liu D, et al. Cyclin D1 genotype, response to biochemoprevention, and progression rate to upper aerodigestive tract cancer. J Natl Cancer Inst 2003;95(3):198–205.
8. Bani-Hani K, Martin IG, Hardie LJ, et al. Prospective study of cyclin D1 overexpression in Barrett's esophagus: association with increased risk of adenocarcinoma. J Natl Cancer Inst 2000;92(16):1316–21.
9. Ye Y, Wang KK, Gu J, et al. Genetic variations in micro RNA-related genes as novel susceptibility loci for esophageal cancer risk. Cancer Prev Res (Phila Pa) 2008;1:460–9.
10. Bild AH, Yao G, Chang JT, et al. Oncogenic pathway signatures in human cancers as a guide to targeted therapies. Nature 2006;439(7074):353–7.
11. Chin L, Gray JW. Translating insights from the cancer genome into clinical practice. Nature 2008;452(7187):553–63.

12. Sawyers CL. The cancer biomarker problem. Nature 2008;452(7187):548–52.
13. van't Veer LJ, Bernards R. Enabling personalized cancer medicine through analysis of gene expression patterns. Nature 2008;452(7187):564–70.
14. Bruzzi JF, Swisher SG, Truong MT, et al. Detection of interval distant metastases: clinical utility of integrated CT-PET imaging in patients with esophageal carcinoma after neoadjuvant therapy. Cancer 2007;109(1):125–34.
15. Erasmus JJ, Munden RF, Truong MT, et al. Preoperative chemoradiation-induced ulceration in patients with esophageal cancer: a confounding factor in tumor response assessment in integrated computed tomographic–positron emission tomographic imaging. J Thorac Oncol 2006;1(5):478–86.
16. Flamen P, Lerut A, Van Cutsem E, et al. Utility of positron emission tomography for the staging of patients with potentially operable esophageal carcinoma. J Clin Oncol 2000;18(18):3202–10.
17. Lordick F, Ott K, Krause BJ, et al. PET to assess early metabolic response and to guide treatment of adenocarcinoma of the oesophagogastric junction: the MUNICON phase II trial. Lancet Oncol 2007;8(9):797–805.
18. Ott K, Herrmann K, Lordick F, et al. Early metabolic response evaluation by fluorine-18 fluorodeoxyglucose positron emission tomography allows in vivo testing of chemosensitivity in gastric cancer: long-term results of a prospective study. Clin Cancer Res 2008;14(7):2012–8.
19. Ott K, Weber W, Siewert JR. The importance of PET in the diagnosis and response evaluation of esophageal cancer. Dis Esophagus 2006;19(6):433–42.
20. Swisher SG, Maish M, Erasmus JJ, et al. Utility of PET, CT, and EUS to identify pathologic responders in esophageal cancer. Ann Thorac Surg 2004;78(4):1152–60 [discussion: 52–60].
21. Weissleder R, Pittet MJ. Imaging in the era of molecular oncology. Nature 2008;452(7187):580–9.
22. Suntharalingam M, Moughan J, Coia LR, et al. The national practice for patients receiving radiation therapy for carcinoma of the esophagus: results of the 1996–1999 Patterns of Care Study. Int J Radiat Oncol Biol Phys 2003;56(4):981–7.
23. Suntharalingam M, Moughan J, Coia LR, et al. Outcome results of the 1996–1999 patterns of care survey of the national practice for patients receiving radiation therapy for carcinoma of the esophagus. J Clin Oncol 2005;23(10):2325–31.
24. Tepper J, Krasna MJ, Niedzwiecki D, et al. Phase III trial of trimodality therapy with cisplatin, fluorouracil, radiotherapy, and surgery compared with surgery alone for esophageal cancer: CALGB 9781. J Clin Oncol 2008;26(7):1086–92.
25. Urba SG, Orringer MB, Turrisi A, et al. Randomized trial of preoperative chemoradiation versus surgery alone in patients with locoregional esophageal carcinoma. J Clin Oncol 2001;19(2):305–13.
26. Bosset JF, Gignoux M, Triboulet JP, et al. Chemoradiotherapy followed by surgery compared with surgery alone in squamous cell cancer of the esophagus. N Engl J Med 1997;337(3):161–7.
27. Walsh TN, Noonan N, Hollywood D, et al. A comparison of multimodal therapy and surgery for esophageal adenocarcinoma. N Engl J Med 1996;335(7):462–7.
28. Ajani JA, Winter K, Komaki R, et al. Phase II randomized trial of two nonoperative regimens of induction chemotherapy followed by chemoradiation in patients with localized carcinoma of the esophagus: RTOG 0113. J Clin Oncol 2008.
29. Kelsen DP, Ginsberg R, Pajak TF, et al. Chemotherapy followed by surgery compared with surgery alone for localized esophageal cancer. N Engl J Med 1998;339(27):1979–84.

30. Chirieac LR, Swisher SG, Ajani JA, et al. Posttherapy pathologic stage predicts survival in patients with esophageal carcinoma receiving preoperative chemora-diation. Cancer 2005;103(7):1347–55.
31. Rohatgi P, Swisher SG, Correa AM, et al. Characterization of pathologic complete response after preoperative chemoradiotherapy in carcinoma of the esophagus and outcome after pathologic complete response. Cancer 2005;104(11): 2365–72.
32. Ajani JA, Correa AM, Swisher SG, et al. For localized gastroesophageal cancer, you give chemoradiation before surgery, but then what happens? J Clin Oncol 2007;25(27):4315–6.
33. Berger AC, Farma J, Scott WJ, et al. Complete response to neoadjuvant chemo-radiotherapy in esophageal carcinoma is associated with significantly improved survival. J Clin Oncol 2005;23(19):4330–7.
34. Rizk NP, Venkatraman E, Bains MS, et al. American Joint Committee on Cancer staging system does not accurately predict survival in patients receiving multimo-dality therapy for esophageal adenocarcinoma. J Clin Oncol 2007;25(5):507–12.
35. Bader FG, Lordick F, Fink U, et al. Paclitaxel in the neoadjuvant treatment for adenocarcinoma of the distal esophagus (AEG I): a comparison of two phase II trials with long-term follow-up. Onkologie 2008;31(7):366–72.
36. Kelsey CR, Chino JP, Willett CG, et al. Paclitaxel-based chemoradiotherapy in the treatment of patients with operable esophageal cancer. Int J Radiat Oncol Biol Phys 2007;69(3):770–6.
37. Javeri H, Arora R, Correa AM, et al. Influence of induction chemotherapy and class of cytotoxics on pathologic response and survival after preoperative che-moradiation in patients with carcinoma of the esophagus. Cancer 2008;113: 1302–8.
38. Hamilton JP, Sato F, Greenwald BD, et al. Promoter methylation and response to chemotherapy and radiation in esophageal cancer. Clin Gastroenterol Hepatol 2006;4(6):701–8.
39. Izzo JG, Malhotra U, Wu TT, et al. Association of activated transcription factor nuclear factor kappab with chemoradiation resistance and poor outcome in esophageal carcinoma. J Clin Oncol 2006;24(5):748–54.
40. Rohatgi PR, Swisher SG, Correa AM, et al. Failure patterns correlate with the proportion of residual carcinoma after preoperative chemoradiotherapy for carci-noma of the esophagus. Cancer 2005;104(7):1349–55.

Index

Note: Page numbers of article titles are in **boldface** type.

A

Acetaldehyde, as risk factor for cancer, 39
Achalasia, as risk factor for cancer, 41
Adenocarcinoma, 60–61
    environmental causes of. *See* Environmental causes.
    epidemiology of, 18
    genetic variations in, 77–83
    prevention of, 68–69
    screening for, 61–63
    surveillance for, 64–68, 183–184
    treatment of. *See* Treatment.
Adjuvant therapy, 139–140
Adult respiratory distress syndrome, after esophagectomy, 175
Africa, epidemiology in, 22
Age factors, in esophageal cancer, 17
Alcohol consumption, as risk factor for cancer, 29, 32, 39
Aldehyde dehydrogenases, polymorphisms of, cancer risk and prognosis and, 79
Anastomotic leak, after esophagectomy, 174–175
Argon plasma coagulation, 127
Asbestos exposure, as risk factor for cancer, 42–43
Asia, epidemiology in, 24
Aspiration pneumonia, after esophagectomy, 175
Aspirin, for cancer prevention, 69
Avenzoar, 6
Avicenna, 4–5

B

Baillie, Matthew, 7
Barrett's esophagus, 60–61
    pathology of
        chemotherapy effects on, 128–131
        histology, 127–128
        muscularis mucosae reduplication, 122–125
        Paget cells, 125–128
        radiation effects on, 128–131
        therapies based on, 126–127
    prevention of, 68–69
    screening for, 61–63
    surveillance for, 64–68, 183–184

Gastroenterol Clin N Am 38 (2009) 189–197
doi:10.1016/S0889-8553(09)00024-7
0889-8553/09/$ – see front matter © 2009 Elsevier Inc. All rights reserved.

gastro.theclinics.com

Moving?

Make sure your subscription moves with you!

To notify us of your new address, find your **Clinics Account Number** (located on your mailing label above your name), and contact customer service at:

E-mail: elspcs@elsevier.com

800-654-2452 (subscribers in the U.S. & Canada)
314-453-7041 (subscribers outside of the U.S. & Canada)

Fax number: 314-523-5170

Elsevier Periodicals Customer Service
11830 Westline Industrial Drive
St. Louis, MO 63146

*To ensure uninterrupted delivery of your subscription, please notify us at least 4 weeks in advance of move.

Printed and bound by CPI Group (UK) Ltd, Croydon, CR0 4YY

03/10/2024

01040443-0001